T0372427

Your Journey, Your Way

Your Journey, Your Way

How to Make the Mental Health System Work for You

HORATIO CLARE

VIKING

an imprint of

PENGUIN BOOKS

VIKING

UK | USA | Canada | Ireland | Australia
India | New Zealand | South Africa

Viking is part of the Penguin Random House group of companies
whose addresses can be found at global.penguinrandomhouse.com.

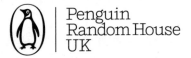

First published 2024
001

Copyright © Horatio Clare, 2024

The moral right of the author has been asserted

Set in 13.5/16pt Garamond MT Std
Typeset by Jouve (UK), Milton Keynes
Printed and bound in Great Britain by Clays Ltd, Elcograf S.p.A.

The authorized representative in the EEA is Penguin Random House Ireland,
Morrison Chambers, 32 Nassau Street, Dublin D02 YH68

A CIP catalogue record for this book is available from the British Library

ISBN: 978–0–241–64133–0

www.greenpenguin.co.uk

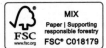

For you, dear reader, in belief and solidarity

Disclaimer

The information in this book has been compiled as general guidance on the specific subjects addressed. It is not a substitute and not to be relied on for medical, healthcare or pharmaceutical professional advice. Please consult your GP before changing, stopping or starting any medical treatment. So far as the author is aware the information given is correct and up to date as at January 2024. Practice, laws and regulations all change and the reader should obtain up-to-date professional advice on any such issues. The author and publishers disclaim, as far as the law allows, any liability arising directly or indirectly from the use or misuse of the information contained in this book.

Contents

ix

CONTENTS

Introduction

This book is for anyone who suffers from mental health troubles, and for anyone who cares for someone who does. Whether your interest is in anxiety or psychosis, clinical depression, insomnia, self-harm, an eating disorder, or any one of many conditions of the mind and brain which can be hell to endure, and hell to witness, you find yourself at a fascinating and dicey moment in how we understand and treat mental health.

The good news is, there is no condition from which we suffer which cannot be helped to some degree, great or small. There are effective treatments – some novel, some established, and many just coming into practice – for pretty well everything. Every sufferer, indeed, every human being, is on a spectrum which runs from very mentally ill to perfectly mentally well, and we do know how to move people along these paths, perhaps a short way, perhaps a significant distance, in a positive direction.

The bad news is that a great many of us, perhaps most of us, do not know which treatments will best suit us – and many of us cannot access the care and support we need. There is a vast amount of information and advice available, but unless you are a specialist professional it can be impossible to know what is accurate, what is relevant and what applies to you. A great deal of what you will find on the internet is outdated, confusing or simply wrong.

This book is a guide to the latest developments in the understanding and treatment of mental health. It explains how to go about helping yourself or someone close to you whom you are worried about. It is journalistic, in that it is accurate, unbiased and has no agenda beyond public service. It explains how mental health treatment models can work and how they can fail, examining their assumptions and mechanisms, and it is written in the certain knowledge that accurate and up-to-date ways of seeing and understanding and treating mental health can really, truly help.

For example, should you read this book before you next meet a doctor, psychiatrist or social worker, you will know something of how they think about you and your condition, what their options are, and how they make their decisions. If you find, having read it, that you know more about what can and might work for you than they do, that should not be surprising. Most practitioners will not know the nuances and specifics of your unique individual condition as well as you do. Most practitioners do not have the time to keep abreast of all the developments in an enormously wide field which spans psychiatry and psychology. Most practitioners do not have access to the leading and most expert researchers and clinicians, whose insights and recommendations are the meat of this book.

Most of us find ourselves caught somewhere between whatever services our local NHS trust can provide (which can be good, or patchy, or inconsistent, or plain inadequate), whatever support we might be able to pay for (i.e. going to a private therapist, assuming one is available, and assuming we can afford one, which many of us cannot), and the infinite uncertainties of whatever we might find on the internet.

This is a hard enough place to be for those of us who are well, and perhaps looking to help and support someone close to us. And it is a truly horrible place to be if you are the one who is suffering. I have been in both of these positions, and to some degree I will always be: I have a mental health condition which needs managing, and I am engaged in trying to help others.

At the end of 2018 I had a breakdown. I was fully, psychotically delusional, believing I was helping the security services and aliens to bring about world peace, and engaged to Kylie Minogue. In the service of world peace I deliberately wrote my car off and started gouging holes in the ceilings of my flat. I was detained under Section 2 of the Mental Health Act and confined to a ward in a psychiatric hospital for a couple of weeks. When I came out, terrified by a choice between a lifetime on medication and a lifetime of worsening madness, I spent days and weeks trawling the internet and books for information and solutions.

Much of what I found was contradicted by other findings. Much turned out to be unsubstantiated. Much was simply wrong. My journalistic interest was piqued.

Over weeks and months my sense of self, my confidence and my powers of research and analysis began to return. I talked to sufferers, families, experts, researchers, practitioners and outliers from across the fields of psychiatry, psychopharmacology, therapy and general medicine, and I found myself, as a journalist, in the middle of what seemed to me a huge and important news story, a story with critical implications for the one in four of us who struggle with our mental health, and for all those who love and worry about us.

For example, did you know that psychiatrists and psychologists are in fundamental disagreement about the causes and best treatments for mental illness? I didn't. Did you know that they even dispute the causes of mental illness? Whole branches of psychiatry assume mental illness has biomedical roots and solutions: the idea that there is something wrong with your brain chemistry. Although neuroscience has yet to find biomarkers in the body or brain which would prove that mental illness is a physical or chemical condition, psychiatry has met much success (and also much failure) by treating people as if the biomedical hypothesis was proved, by prescribing chemicals.

Meanwhile, whole areas of psychology believe the questions and answers to mental distress do not lie in physical brain deformities or in the balance of chemicals in the brain. Psychology believes that the troubles, and the answers, most often lie in the sufferer's context, i.e. in your life history and personal circumstances.

Psychiatry points to the huge numbers of people who have been helped, even saved, by psychiatric medication. Psychology and critics of psychiatry, including many sufferers and their families, point to the huge numbers of people who have not been helped by psychiatric drugs, and those who have suffered for taking them.

I was amazed to find that psychiatry and psychology do not even agree on the language and terminology of mental health. Psychiatry talks about 'mental illness' and about 'disorders'. Psychology talks about 'distress' and 'sufferers'. Many psychiatrists – and certainly two of the three who have treated me – assume that disorders are located in the brain (the other one was French; she saw my situation differently, and had very different solutions to it). Many psychologists see childhood and life events as the place to look for and address the problem. How, I wondered, are we going to solve or salve mental illness and suffering if we cannot agree where it comes from, what to call it, or how to treat it?

Like many people who know what they want to find – for me, a third way, a way out of the crushing binary choice of long-term drugs or madness – I set about looking for it in ways which seemed most likely to deliver it. I read much more literature from the anti-psychiatry side of the debate than from the pro-psychiatry side, and listened carefully to those – including many psychiatrists – who question or condemn the way things are now.

This was partly defiance and partly panic. I was under heavy pressure to accept the diagnosis two psychiatrists had given me – bipolar – and to take lithium or aripiprazole or another antipsychotic for years, perhaps for life. I was not looking for the most effective way out, necessarily: I was looking for a way of being sane while not taking long-term drugs; for a way of being normal, or at least balanced, in ways the bipolar diagnosis did not seem to offer, unless I took the drugs. It turns out, as I found, that there is no basic right or wrong with psychiatric drugs. They can do enormous, lifesaving good, and they can do great harm. What you really need, and what you are most unlikely to get, is deep specialist knowledge of how you might best move forward according to the most up-to-date thinking in understanding your condition, in the use of psychiatric drugs, in actions you can take, in therapy and in recovery pathways. You will find that knowledge and that thinking here.

After years of research and asking questions I found ways forward for me, and I found that they exist, to a greater or lesser extent, for all of us. I do not mean we can all be healed, or that we can all reach a place of total recovery, but I absolutely do mean and have found that we can all be made better than we are. This book will not make false or exaggerated promises. It is a guide to the ways in which healing happens; it is a map of the paths to recovery that researchers and practitioners and sufferers know about and are exploring.

We cannot be made better unless we are well informed.

We cannot be made better without taking significant action. We cannot be made better without making changes to our lives. We cannot be made better without help and support. We cannot be made better without the fullest possible understanding of our conditions, both their general shape and kind, and the precise and individual ways in which they play out in us. We cannot be made better without understanding the mental health treatment system that we find ourselves in. We cannot be made better without distinguishing between what is happening to us and who we are.

Researching the story and the landscape of mental health treatment was healing in itself – finding meaningful activities and interests is a key part of recovery, as we will see – and writing about it even more so. The book I published in 2020, *Heavy Light: A Journey through Madness, Mania & Healing*, describes the small but intense story of my own breakdown, and reports on the states, as I found them, of psychiatry's and psychology's understanding, ignorance and methods. It tells how, through privilege (white, male, middle-class, relatively moneyed privilege), persistence and good fortune, I found my third way; or at least the start of a path of ongoing recovery.

Broadly, psychiatry finds the first part of my story valid and useful, in its lucid descriptions and reports from inside a state of psychotic delusion. Social workers and other professionals in the field of mental health find the view of the system from the inside telling and illuminating. Sufferers and those close to them find hope and inspiration in the second part, in the story of how you can define your own terms, personalise and hone your own diagnosis, and how you can research and design your own treatment plan.

My own family and I find the book flawed, in retrospect, in that it tells two parts of a three-part story. Missing from *Heavy Light* is what happened after that book ends, in the changes and adjustments I and my family made to how we lived in the light of all that we and I had learned. Salman Rushdie once wrote that books find people to write them. I would never have chosen to go through – never mind put my family through – the experiences which gave me *Heavy Light*. But I am very grateful that I was able to make a book out of them, and I am very grateful that by living out that story and that book, my family and I were able to move to a better, stronger, richer place. But the thing is, when you send a book out into the world it grabs you by the hand and takes you with it, which is how we come to *Your Journey, Your Way*.

Touring *Heavy Light* and talking about it, I soon found myself in a widening and deepening conversation with readers, audiences and correspondents, many of whom are professionals, about what we do and do not know about mental health, and how we should and should not treat it. This led to two BBC Radio 4 series of *Is Psychiatry Working?* which I wrote and co-presented with a wonderfully expert and eminent psychiatrist, a true star in his field, Professor Femi Oyebode of the University of Birmingham.

From Femi and from our dozens of interviewees – who ranged from the President of the Royal College of Psychiatrists to respected academics and practitioners who oppose many of psychiatry's practices and deny its fundamental tenets – I saw something of the breadth of our understandings of mental health and how to help it. I began to comprehend something of the depth of the field's complexity: the human brain remains one of the more intricate and mysterious creations in the known universe.

Most inspiringly and most urgently, I gained insight into the ways in which the people of the near future, our children and grandchildren, may be supported or let down by how we think about mental health, and what we do about it.

And that is how this book found me, and this is why I felt, very strongly, that it needed to be written. Because most people who suffer, and most people who care for us, and, strikingly, a great many people who are paid to treat us and care for us, do not know or are only vaguely aware of what the latest findings and treatments are.

This book will tell you everything I have found and learned about this vital subject. I wrote it because it insisted I write it, out of a sense of outrage at the disastrous ways we misunderstand and mistreat people who suffer from mental ill health, and out of hope and excitement at the prospect of new models of treatment and the good they can and will do.

The evidence is clear that, together, treatments like Open Dialogue, Eye Movement Desensitisation and Reprocessing (EMDR) and the recovery model can and will change the world for many, many people (see Chapter 19). Our understanding of mental health is imperfect and developing all the time, and so this book is imperfect, describing the beginnings and early adoptions of treatments and ways of seeing which are bound to become clearer, more influential and more widespread. But this book is also honest and accurate. I hope you find something in it that is helpful to you: I really, deeply hope that.

One more thing: I wrote a good chunk of this book when I was miserable and scared, plugging through my usual winter blues in Yorkshire. So if you are in a hard mental place, now, then we're in it together. Hang in there. Things really can and will get better. This book shows how that can happen, and I wrote it for you.

1. Ways of thinking and talking about what is happening to you

To begin at the beginning, let us imagine you are in trouble. In the West today, general medical practice is, first, to identify as accurately and quickly as we can what sort of trouble you are in. Because mental distress does not show up on a blood test, or a brain scan, an X-ray or on any kind of system of technological measurement, we do this by asking you questions, by looking at what we can of your medical history, your past and current circumstances, by talking to those close to you (where possible and appropriate), and by coming up with a description of your position.

Can't sleep? *Insomnia.* Distressed and nervous? *Anxiety.* Persistent low mood, unhappy, feeling worthless, guilty, suicidal? *Depression.*

We do not spend much time worrying about niceties of language. You are not likely to be described as 'temporarily depressed', or 'experiencing insomnia': instead, you are likely to be diagnosed as depressed or insomniac or anxious – suffering from depressive disorder, or anxiety disorder, or a sleep disorder, et cetera.

But notice that there are two things at work here. Are you depressed at the moment, or are you someone who suffers from depression? Are you experiencing, due to life events, an understandable period of insecurity, which is making you anxious and miserable, or do you have an anxiety disorder? Do you actually suffer from a sleep disorder, or are you temporarily in the grip of insomnia?

I have found it very useful to separate the two; dividing the experience (say, insomnia) from the diagnosis (a sleep disorder). I have had periods of depression, and several of them made me want to die – not to kill myself (though I thought about suicide a lot), but rather, to not exist at all. According to medical criteria, I could identify as a depressive, someone who suffers with a depressive disorder, which I could see as part of me – as who I am.

But I don't. Most of my depressions were associated with a withdrawal from cannabis, and almost all happened in the winter. All of them were strongly associated with unhappy life situations: in university, later at work, or at home, or both. I conclude, therefore, that I do not have a depressive disorder: rather, if I smoke dope and then stop, or if my personal or professional life is not making me happy, I get depressed.

You might find you are suffering from anxiety which is particularly triggered by situations at work (like going to work when miserable – I've sure had that) or at home. But does this mean there is something wrong with your brain? No, it absolutely does not. Science has never come close to identifying a brain deformity or malfunction associated with anxiety. Does it mean you have a disorder? Well, it *might* mean you are a sensitive, perhaps naturally anxious person with what seems to be a chronic condition. And so, yes, that could be described as a disorder. But it is also perfectly possible, isn't it, that the pressures on you at work, or your situation at home, are making you horribly anxious? In which case your reaction is not just understandable, it is normal, even healthy. Your anxiety might be your gut instinct telling you to leave that job, or find ways of doing it differently, or change your life at home.

The fact is, your brain, mind and body are not the same as the brain, mind and body of anyone else on earth. This means that your depression or anxiety or insomnia are not the same as anyone else's, either. They may present as very similar, but they are not the same. So – as a unique individual – you have (however subtle the differences) unique troubles.

Every doctor, psychiatrist, therapist and scientist on earth would agree that your troubles, and your brain, mind and body need to be helped, treated and supported in a unique way, personalised to you. The problem is, unless you are very wealthy and prepared to go private, the system we have does not have the time, money or resources to do that. You will be treated in more or less the same way as people who have more or less similar presentations. (And even if you do have the money and are going to go private, as we will see, you will still need to be lucky and in possession of a lot of relevant, quite specialist knowledge if you are going to get the treatment you need.)

By 'presentations' we mean how you appear, and what you say about how you are feeling, and what you have been experiencing. So when you meet any clinician, from a nurse to a consultant psychiatrist, it is worth being as detailed and accurate and honest as you can about how you are feeling, what you think might be causing it, your life circumstances, et cetera. You must not rush or hold back, if at all possible. We will come back to this.

Experience and research have taught me that it is really helpful to remember – and, when appropriate, make a noise about – the uniqueness of your own mental troubles. It helps you get the best, most personalised treatment.

And so this is my rule number one, and I would like you to consider making use of it, in case it helps. I am *not* saying it will work for everyone, but for me, this is it:

Rule 1: No one else has what I have.

Millions of people worldwide go through very similar suffering, with near identical symptoms. But it helps me to remember that my symptoms are specific to me, and arose from my experience of the world, my life circumstances, jobs and relationships, perhaps from my genes, definitely from things that happened to me and things that I did or did not do.

I find that thinking like this allows me a sense of freedom and control, which helps me manage my ups and downs.

If, on the other hand, it would give me comfort and

strength to identify as someone who suffers from a depressive disorder, in solidarity with millions who also identify this way, then I definitely *would* identify that way.

Sometimes I do, in that I sometimes say, 'I am seasonally affective,' or 'I have Seasonal Affective Disorder.' SAD is a condition in which sufferers feel depressed, with low mood, low energy, low self-esteem, low hope (in my case) and high anxiety in the winter months. SAD's changes in mood and behaviour (including sleeping too much or too little, and gorging on high-fat, high-sugar foods) seem to be linked to day length, exposure to sunlight and possibly vitamin D deficiency. Researchers identified the condition by comparing the experiences of winter shared by people living in the northern, darker and colder regions of the United States with the sunny winter experiences of people living in Florida.

I have found this diagnosis a helpful shorthand. (No doctor has given it to me – they don't need to. I get the blues on about November 11th every year, and start coming out around January 11th.) It's helpful when I am dragging my miserable carcass through the daily tasks, school run, work, food shop, feeling dark, and I run into a friend who can see I'm down. 'It's just SAD,' I say, 'I'm seasonally affective,' and many people now know roughly what that means, and so we are both reassured. My family are familiar with it, too, and while they are sympathetic they are unalarmed by it: we all know I will come through. Identifying with the diagnosis also encourages me to take steps to fight the blues in the winter (with

SAD lamps, exercise, vitamins, diet, et cetera). But here is the crucial point: *I decide what I have, and what to call it. No one else.* If I found it stigmatising, or inaccurate, or in any way unhelpful, I would ditch it.

But, I hear you say, doesn't the language of diagnosis, of what I've got, belong to the doctors, psychiatrists and the researchers? Isn't it up to medical science to identify my symptoms and say what I have? Well, yes – and no. The thing to note is, the science of mental distress is (and frankly admits it is) inexact, and overwhelmingly based on hypotheses. In other words, the language, diagnoses and descriptions that professionals use are not definitive fact so much as *the nearest we can come to the truth*, based on what we know in a constantly developing field.

So, your leg is either broken – a fracture of the tibia, say – or it is not. But in mental health, you might be having a single episode of what we describe as depression (you could call it a bite of the Black Dog, or a reaction to trauma, or a bad attack of the blues), or you might be manifesting symptoms that meet the criteria of what is described as a depressive disorder. So suppose someone you love dies. You go through grief. That might last weeks, months or years. But according to one influential diagnostic manual, the *Diagnostic and Statistical Manual of Mental Disorders*, which is used widely by psychiatrists in America, if your grief lasts longer than a year, for adults, or six months for children, you have Prolonged Grief Disorder.

Now, what is going to help you recover and live well: believing you are naturally and normally grieving your loved one, or believing you have Prolonged Grief Disorder? In my case, I am still grieving for my sister, who died in 2011, and my father, who died in 2019. Do I believe I have Prolonged Grief Disorder? Do I hell. And so I don't have to add that disorder to a list of other things, like SAD and cyclothymia (a mild form of bipolar, barely known in the UK, with which I was diagnosed by a doctor I trusted in France), which I do think I suffer from. So in this case, I have literally thought and decided my way out of a diagnosis I think is bogus. You cannot do that with a broken leg. You cannot think or act your leg into being unbroken, and whatever you do or do not do, broken it is. But how you think about your experience of mental struggle, and what actions you take, will absolutely, definitely and deeply affect and change what happens to your condition and to you.

2. Who owns the words?
(And why they matter)

So if it can be rather uncertain, this diagnosis business, what is the role of the doctor and the psychiatrist? How much weight should you give what they tell you? Well, whether you have a broken leg or the blues, our system is designed so that a typical appointment with a doctor lasts fifteen minutes. In that time, the doctor – who *may* be very brilliant, very experienced, very up on the latest developments in the field of (say) depression, and very interested in you – will have to establish your current state and symptoms, your history of symptoms, something of your circumstances, and gather information on any life events or other afflictions which may have a bearing on your situation.

The doctor will then aim to come up with a diagnosis, which in turn implies some options for treatment, and advice. They may well refer you to a psychiatrist, or recommend you look at the availability of therapy, or both. They may prescribe medication.

Doctors and psychiatrists wish to treat you as an individual, of course, but they lack the therapist's relative luxury of time. So the accepted practice is to place you, as quickly and accurately as possible, in the category that best seems to describe someone with your symptoms, grouping you with all those people whose condition is most like yours. It is a sensible process, given the pressure our systems are under.

However, the categories in which you are placed (in Britain) come from a manual called the *International Classification of Diseases*. The part dealing with mental health and well-being is based on the *Diagnostic and Statistical Manual of Mental Disorders*, an American publication drawn up by the American Psychiatric Association. The *DSM*, as it is known, is made up of checklists of symptoms which it matches with diagnoses.

A part of the training of the doctor or psychiatrist who is about to diagnose your disorder is memorising these checklists. Some disorders only require two of twenty different symptoms to be present, so five people suffering two different symptoms each all come away with one and the same diagnosis. So supposing I am exhibiting 'disorganised speech' (which would come across as random or ranting or both) and loss of interest in the world ('negative symptoms') and catatonia (I can barely get out of bed). And suppose you are suffering delusions (you believe you are working for aliens on their world peace project) and hallucinations (you are seeing things, like that massive pink butterfly sitting on top of your flatmate's head, which are not actually there). According to diagnostic criteria, we are both schizophrenic.

Is that useful to us? Are we really suffering from the same problems, with the same causes? In fact, how and why people develop schizophrenia are mysteries. As the NHS puts it, 'The exact causes of schizophrenia are unknown. Research suggests a combination of physical, genetic, psychological and environmental factors can make a person more likely to develop the condition.' So, with our differing symptoms, should we be treated with the same drugs, as we will be?

My point is that, although they may be very useful, and certainly help and treat many millions of people, diagnoses are not an exact science. In the case of schizophrenia many practising and academic psychiatrists, alongside sociologists and historians of psychiatry, now believe that the schizophrenia diagnosis will end up being scrapped, leading to the reclassification of its symptoms as various forms of psychosis.

Strictly speaking, diagnoses are not a science so much as a series of descriptions. This is because you cannot point to mental illnesses on an MRI scan or see them under a microscope; they do not physically exist. The acclaimed psychiatrist, my co-presenter on our two Radio 4 series, Professor Femi Oyebode, puts it like this: '[Mental] diseases are merely concepts. In other words, they aren't things but ideas about how to organise the world.'

And so it is worth thinking long and hard about how well and specifically you were able to describe your situation, your history and your symptoms to your clinician.

And think about how closely your clinician listened.

And consider how carefully, subtly and individually, he, she or they thought about what your diagnosis should be.

Because – here's a surprise – although, after repeated episodes, the brains of depressed, manic, delusional or psychotic people may show marginal differences from 'normal' brains, the margins are so small as to be scientifically and practically useless. 'We cannot look into *your* brain,' a consultant psychiatrist told me.

If you have a brain tumour, we can scan you and see it. If you have any form of mental distress, we can scan you as much as we like – but we cannot tell your brain apart from any other normal brain.*

This is why the language of distress is so important. For example:

At the end of the nineteenth century a woman who went from dazzling optimism to profound gloom to loss of touch with reality would have been diagnosed, according to the descriptive criteria of the time, with hysteria, or a nervous breakdown.

If she had been in the trenches of the First World War, she would have been diagnosed with shell shock.

In the later twentieth century she would have been diagnosed with manic depression.

---

* We do know that people who have suffered from and been treated for conditions like psychosis and schizophrenia may show a degree of brain damage, in the form of changes to basal ganglion structures, the thalamus and frontal lobes. The worry is that MRI studies have shown these changes can be caused by antipsychotic medication.

Now, today, she would be diagnosed with bipolar disorder, with possible post-traumatic stress disorder (PTSD) and, depending on how she behaved and which clinicians she encountered, possibly a borderline personality disorder, too.

So the same woman, with the same symptoms, experiencing the same suffering, would get different diagnoses and different treatments.

Of course medicine and science advance, and language changes with them. But the words and the language we used to diagnose this time-travelling woman at each stage of her journey led to her having different treatments and being perceived in different ways. In turn, the words and the language we used affected how she thought and felt about what she was going through, what she *was* (a hysteric, a bipolar sufferer, et cetera), and this had a huge influence over the actions she took and the life changes she did or did not make. And so although she suffers from the same things at each stage, as a direct consequence of the language used, her outcomes and her life experiences are widely, wildly different.

The worry is that the evidence suggests this woman's chances of recovery, remission, or healing are no higher now than they were a century ago. In fact, some researchers believe they are worse. As the journalist and author Robert Whitaker points out, before the modern era, including the drug treatments which changed psychiatric treatment from the 1950s onwards, in cases of what was then called manic depression, now bipolar disorder,

'85 percent of bipolar patients would regain complete functioning and return to work'. Now only a third achieve 'full social and occupational functional recovery'. He cites a 2007 study by Nancy Huxley, Assistant Professor of Psychiatry at Harvard, and Ross J. Baldessarini, Professor of Psychiatry at Harvard, both internationally respected career-long specialists in bipolar disorder, which concludes: 'Prognosis for bipolar disorder was once considered relatively favorable, but contemporary findings suggest that disability and poor outcomes are prevalent, despite major therapeutic advances.'

It is worth noting that Robert Whitaker, as well as being a journalist, is a well-known campaigner against the over-prescription (by which he means a significant level of prescriptions, even the majority of prescriptions) of psychiatric drugs. But although his conclusions are disputed, the integrity of his research and findings are unquestioned – indeed, they are award-winning.

Psychiatry states that we can and do help vastly more people in vastly better ways than we did, thanks to drug treatments. But for certain conditions we have not gone forwards. For example, people who suffered nervous breakdowns at the turn of the twentieth century had similar or better rates of recovery than do people who experience one today. Conclusions are hard to draw, but language and expectation certainly play a vital role. Being told, for example, 'You have had a breakdown,' in a social context like the early twentieth century, where breakdowns are not uncommon, and many people recover from them, is a very different experience (and invites different treatment) from being told, 'You have bipolar disorder,' (a lifetime condition with no cure).

So my rule number two is:

Rule 2: I call it whatever is most helpful to me.

For example, presenting the same set of symptoms, I was diagnosed with cyclothymia in France, and bipolar in the UK. Having had no reoccurrence in four years, I conclude either:

a) the bipolar diagnosis was wrong (I ought to have had more and more severe episodes by now, according to the criteria, but I haven't), or

b) I am 'in remission', or

c) the criteria and diagnoses that we have only partly describe what I have, and are only therefore partly useful to me.

Yes, I've gone for c.

As it happens, one psychiatrist said I had cyclothymia – as you will recall from the book's introduction, a rarer and milder form of bipolar – two psychiatrists said bipolar, and two psychotherapists advised I dump the labels entirely, as they do not find it helpful in treatment. Neither did I. So now I do not identify as bipolar, but rather as someone who had a breakdown. I believe I had a breakdown for very clear reasons, produced by underlying conditions laid down in childhood, and my subsequent actions, behaviour and circumstances. I do go up and down (happier in summer, lower in winter); I can definitely reach a hypomanic pitch if I smoke dope, work too hard, stay up too late and drink too much, but these are a world away from a breakdown. I do not fear another breakdown, because I put effort into changing my circumstances, and changing my actions and behaviour.

If you were to take this path, then you would have to accept that many experts, including extremely eminent psychiatrists of impeccable integrity and vast experience, would shake their heads and conclude you are in some sort of denial.

At the same time, no doctor or psychiatrist who is any good at all would seek to deny or disprove or even debate your choice, if they judged it was helpful to you, because professional healers and competent clinicians are all in favour of whatever works for the patient.

So, to sum up: I believe I am a good example of how choosing your own language is really helpful. I found that after all my personal experience and subsequent research, listening to professional opinions while holding on to the knowledge that no one is ever going to know my circumstances and my symptoms better than I do has made me more certain about and less worried by my mental health. Researching and thinking about and drawing up my own, personalised understanding of and terminology for what I have been through (and what I will go through, no doubt) has made *all* the difference to my life, and huge positive differences to the lives of those closest to me.

But what is important here is what works for you. A writer I respect very much, as a person and an artist, announced at the beginning of a creative writing course I lead that she has bipolar. She explained this might mean she missed sessions, gave me and her peers to understand she was taking medication which had side effects, and gave us all the impression that though bipolar was a serious part of her life, it was nothing to be ashamed or scared of; she was dedicated to managing it; she might require our support.

Of course she got our support. The experience of her openness was doubly wonderful because the whole group felt we had a responsibility to repay her frankness and courage with our understanding. And we could all see that the diagnosis she owned and the treatment she was undergoing for it were working for her.

We admired her courage and strength. When she did not turn up to sessions we sympathised. When she got very high marks we were delighted but not surprised: she took the same courage and energy to her work. She is a perfect example of the opposite approach from mine succeeding.

It is also worth knowing about another writer, a highly successful poet and teacher. We did an event together in a small northern town, in the rain, in winter, on a dark night during a fuel strike, on the lurking edge of the pandemic. She is a tremendous, powerful presence and truly outstanding poet and performer. We discussed our diagnoses. She has a resonant and mighty voice, and in it she said, 'They told me I had borderline personality disorder. I said, "No, fuck that. I'm a poet." And I have been ever since.'

3. What I've got: Diagnosis (just for you)

Diagnoses: pros and cons
Pros

1. Having a diagnosis may help you, your family, friends, colleagues and employers gain insight into your situation, and help you gather support.
2. Having a diagnosis can be extremely helpful in professional and legal situations – for example, in relation to employment law.
3. Having a diagnosis will entitle you to treatment, possibly including medication.
4. Having a diagnosis can be hugely personally comforting – a feeling of, 'At last, I know what the trouble is!'
5. Having a diagnosis may give you ways to understand your troubles, to explore, research and manage them in the individual ways that suit you best.
6. Having a diagnosis allows health-care systems, from the NHS to charitable institutions and support groups, to identify and appreciate your condition efficiently and quickly provide you with help and support.

7. In terms of health insurance, a diagnosis can make all the difference. You may need a diagnosis in order to access funding for treatment (this is especially true in the United States).
8. The criteria for diagnoses and the treatment for identified conditions are evolving. Being diagnosed and being part of the health system may allow you to keep up with the latest thinking and access the latest treatments.

Cons

1. The diagnosis may be wrong.
2. Diagnosis 'ends curiosity in the system', as one senior and team-leading NHS therapist put it: clinicians may treat you according to the diagnosis, rather than treating you individually.
3. Diagnosis can bring stigma: one psychiatrist I know says many people in his large catchment of patients in South London experience the stigma of being known to have a mental health condition as worse than the condition. Bad enough that you are bipolar, for example, but perhaps you can handle that in ways you cannot handle people judging you because you are known to be 'mental'. Perhaps you are known to have been sectioned. Suppose you have kids, and they have to put up with stuff about you in the playground . . . I still find it uncomfortable,

sometimes, to watch and sense the reaction of someone when I tell them I was sectioned. Much worse, for me, were the years before I got and dealt with the diagnosis, and worried that I was bipolar. The massive stigma I was absolutely terrified of was the stigma I was going to get for being 'a nutter with a disorder' from *me*.

4. Diagnosis can cause feelings of despair and hopelessness: if you are diagnosed with a lifetime condition, you may feel you have no way out, no way back to being normal / healthy / free of the condition / well.

5. Diagnoses often imply medication, but mental health medication is not an exact science. Psychiatric medication is prescribed by trial and error, and adjusted according to the effects and side effects you report. Although medication can be a lifesaver, especially in acute crisis, being prescribed the wrong medication or too much medication can, and does, do harm.

6. The criteria for diagnosis are inexact and they change. Homosexuality was a diagnosable disorder until 1973. In 2022, there was uproar when the 5th edition of the *Diagnostic and Statistical Manual of Mental Disorders* designated grief lasting more than twelve months as a diagnosable disorder. Of *DSM 5* the renowned psychiatrist Allen Frances, who chaired the task

force which published the 4th edition, said, 'Don't buy it, don't teach it.'

7. You may find you suffer, or your suffering changes, in ways the diagnosis does not account for. So suppose you have been diagnosed with borderline personality disorder. But then your life circumstances change, and two years on you find you are no longer so anxious, so insecure about your friendships, and not suffering mood swings or losing your temper as you were before. Do you still have borderline personality disorder? Has it changed into something else? Did you ever have it?

8. In mental health, a diagnosis is given when you manifest certain symptoms within a general descriptive category: it is not a specific-to-you, final truth.

Having spoken to countless experts and having experienced both extremely positive and scarily negative effects of diagnoses, I remain in favour of getting a diagnosis – although how much notice you take of it is up to you, and really worth thinking about.

So here's my diagnosis story in more detail. In France, during a hot summer which I celebrated with cannabis, alcohol, overexcited partying and no sleep, I ended up in hospital being interviewed by a psychiatrist. She was a remarkable woman, who specialised in war trauma, among other fields. After posing questions about my state and my circumstances, she asked me what I thought might be happening to me.

I said, 'I think I am bipolar, and I think I'm having an attack.'

She said, 'Well, that can't be right.'

'Why not?'

'Because you wouldn't be able to have this conversation with me.'

I was flummoxed. I said, 'So what is wrong with me?'

'You have cyclothymia,' she said.

I had never heard of cyclothymia.

'It is like a rare, mild form of bipolar,' she explained. 'You can go up, you can go down. It can get better or it can get worse. There is no cure, but if you are careful, you can manage it.'

She gave me a packet of pills – loxapine, an antipsychotic – and told me that if I found myself staying up too late, becoming manic, doing too much or talking too fast, I should take one. It would help me sleep and calm me down, she said.

It worked. Occasionally, I would find myself taking one: it would make me feel a bit stoned until I made it to my bed, whereupon I would fall into a deep, deep sleep, and wake feeling and acting sane and steady.

Big personal thumbs up for diagnosis and medication, in this case.

And the wonderful thing was, when I looked up cyclothymia on the internet, it seemed to describe me perfectly – better, more accurately, than 'bipolar' had ever seemed to do. I cannot tell you how relieved and glad I was to have that diagnosis. I was not mad or weird or lost – I was cyclothymic! I told my family and my closest friends. Everyone seemed relieved – or at least, happy to see me relieved.

However, some years later, after a busy autumn and early winter which I celebrated with (wait for it) waaay too much cannabis, alcohol, overexcited partying and no sleep, I had my full-on psychotic breakdown and ended up sectioned in a mental hospital in Wakefield, under the care (and total power) of a psychiatrist. He told me I was bipolar. I said I thought I was seasonally affective, vulnerable to cannabis psychosis, and suffering from cyclothymia.

'All this is bipolar,' he said, rather dismissively.

It turns out that while cyclothymia is a relatively rare diagnosis in Britain, it is well known and commonly diagnosed in France, where it is also known as Bipolar Type 2.5, or 'soft bipolar'. Large-scale studies into degrees of bipolar, including cyclothymia, have been carried out in France, where four regional centres are being funded and dedicated to studying the subtleties and best treatments for the hugely varied range of individual conditions currently lumped together as 'bipolar'. (For what it's worth, I bet fifty quid that the whole 'bipolar' diagnosis will be gone in ten years' time, replaced with a spectrum of more nuanced descriptions. Or, I bet they will be in France, anyway.) Startling claims have been made for cyclothymia: taking issue with the

DSM 5's assessment that cyclothymia is a subtype of Bipolar Disorder 1, Giulio Perugi and his fellow researchers published a paper in 2015 asserting:

> Data emerging from both academic centers and from public and private outpatient facilities indicate that from 20% to 50% of all subjects that seek help for mood, anxiety, impulsive and addictive disorders turn out, after careful screening, to be affected by cyclothymia.

The moral of this little story is the moral of this book: it is vital to research, explore and take ownership of your subtle, unique and individual condition, and it is vital to take great care that you are not undermined, misled or damaged by labels which can be clumsy – leading to treatments which can be unhelpful or harmful.

Although I agreed that my symptoms met official diagnostic criteria for the condition psychiatrists call 'bipolar', I stood by my own assessment of what I had – cyclothymia, SAD, drug and alcohol issues, a failing relationship, deep self-loathing brought on by (and enabling) cheating on my partner and lying to her, and huge work pressures, leading to a psychotic episode which was partly due to sleep deprivation and significantly to cannabis, powerful strains of which make me manic.

So it was that I found the psychiatrist's 'all this is bipolar' diagnosis, and the life-changing pills he wanted me to take, unconvincing to the point of terrifying and undermining. So far, five years, give or take, later, time has shown I was right and the diagnosis was wrong.

If I was classic bipolar I should have had another and worse breakdown by now. I haven't. I should have gone raging high and plunging low. I haven't. (Although a SAD low feels utterly awful, it is not as bad as clinical depression. It feels like hell, sometimes, but it's worth remembering that even hell has a shallow end.) I have been summer up and winter down, and I continue to manage this cyclothymic cycle.

My GP (who is the practice mental health lead – an important point for any sufferer, to which we shall return) tells me that his practice designates people as 'in remission' from bipolar after five years of no psychiatric drugs and no help from clinical services. As I write this, I am five months off that official 'remission' point. As you read it – fingers really crossed – I should be months or years past it.

Had I taken long-term antipsychotic medication, as my psychiatrist wanted me to, I am absolutely sure I would have struggled to keep it up. I would certainly have missed doses and I have no private doubt that I would have tried to discontinue it by quitting, going cold turkey. The evidence is unambiguous that had I done so, my outcomes would have been as bad as or worse than those of an unmedicated bipolar sufferer. (Indeed, there is mounting evidence from the longest studies that for many people, long-term antipsychotic use is more harmful than never taking them. If you are taking long-term medication and it is working for you then you are NOT one of these people. You are doing the right thing for you, and I salute you.)

But, the upshot of this story is a big personal thumbs down for diagnosis and medication, in this case.

Conclusion? Well, I feel it is worth getting a diagnosis, of course. It may – it *should* – lead to serious changes in a positive direction. It is worth getting as many opinions as possible. But do think about what you have read here, the pros and cons. A diagnosis may be the best thing that could possibly happen to you, and lead to actions or treatments that hugely improve your life. Or a diagnosis may be wrong, or undermining, or unhelpful, or even devastating, and lead to actions and treatments which do not help, or even worsen, your life.

Either way, you are what matters, not what *anyone else* thinks or says. I know people who have had to really fight to get a diagnosis, and when they got it, found it was so helpful as to be life-changing. Equally, I know people who have experienced diagnosis as disastrous, and have had to really fight the consequences.

When I talk to people who have had diagnoses, I ask: Does having that diagnosis help you sleep at night? Does it make you feel better about the world and more hopeful about your life? If so, keep it. But if it doesn't, if it scares you or worries you, you might think about dumping it, and coming up with your own.

In the end, no one else is you: there has never been a you before and there never will be again, and there is no cure or pill for being you. There might well be medication for your symptoms, which really works and

26

changes your life for the better. But you are not your symptoms.

You may be experiencing insomnia, anxiety, depression, delusion, psychosis, mania, anhedonia, grief, love, obsession, loneliness, ecstasy, trauma or fear, or any other kind of struggle. But you are not these things. You are not your suffering.

Rule 3: I am not my suffering; I am not my symptoms.

My strategy is to think of mental suffering as a kind country I am travelling through. It is a country that many of us travel through, in our own ways. When I am in it, I try to keep telling myself that this may be a hard and scary country now, but the trick is to keep travelling, and to see if I can find ways to make the journey easier.

4. Don't believe the hype

There is a serious worry which is shared by doctors, psychiatrists, psychotherapists, and many people outside the medical and therapeutic systems, especially parents and friends of sufferers, concerning the internet, diagnoses and self-diagnoses.

The first thing most of us do, when trouble of any kind comes, is look it up online. For medical professionals, from general practitioners to consultants (and including clinicians and therapists of every kind), the sufferer sitting in their office with a self-made diagnosis from Google is a fact of modern life. It is a lot easier (seconds) to get an appointment and diagnosis from the internet than it is to get an appointment with a doctor (days or weeks), a psychiatrist (weeks or months) or a therapist (days or weeks, if you can afford to go private, months if you cannot).

In mental health this is an issue because:

- A diagnosis from a website, though it may have no clinical basis, may seem to carry the weight of fact: that 'Aha, that's me / That's what I've got!' feeling.
- Self-diagnosis can change – including dramatically for the worse – a sufferer's

behaviour, beliefs, fears and sense of hope and possibility.

- Self-diagnosis is often received in isolation (in that private space between you and your phone or laptop) with no one to discuss it with, no second or qualified opinion, and no human, real-world support.
- Young people especially (everyone below the age of forty is 'young' for the purposes of this book) suffer from internet self-diagnosis, because young people spend more time on the web, are more at home with it, are more likely to trust it, and are less practised and familiar with accessing doctors and appropriate NHS services than are older and wealthier generations.
- People who are not well off, not white and not privileged within society are much more likely to end up in A&E and are much less likely to find a path to the specialist medical treatment that would most benefit them: a phone and a search engine is often their key – indeed, their only practical and available – resource.
- Children and young adults who are naturally finding their way and exploring possibilities of being and identity may attach disproportionate, all-consuming weight to a self-diagnosis.

A model which is familiar to many clinicians, parents and teachers and lecturers runs:

I am anxious (for example) – google it.

Looks like I have anxiety disorder – google it.

Anxiety disorder can have severe effects on an individual's life and behaviour – google it.

Find more symptoms which I may or may not have.

Brood over those I may have.

Decide my anxiety has serious effects on my life and behaviour. Act accordingly; including online.

My identity and my anxiety disorder become strongly, or inextricably linked.

I have become my anxiety: I feel scared, and, if challenged, perhaps defensive, certainly isolated – *and ever more anxious.*

I may need/want/experiment with medication and/or self-medication.

I may avoid social situations; I may withdraw into a largely online life.

Result: I have made my anxious situation much worse.

Rule 4: No website can know me better than I can know myself.

There is a good side to the availability of information on the internet, of course. The psychiatrist Matthew Broome, who specialises in working with children and young people at the University of Birmingham, told me that he found young people are very well informed about the possibilities of what they might be suffering from, and do not shy away from mental health diagnoses or treatment in the way that older people from previous generations might have done. Growing up in a culture which is more open about mental illness than it was, and with more information available, can make the young more ready to accept and tackle mental conditions, and less vulnerable to stigma.

This is in no way intended to minimise the hell that is suffering when you are young. I found my first experiences of anxiety and depression in my early twenties utterly terrifying. I did not know I would come through them; I had no experiences of resilience and recovery to draw upon. It did not make any difference that other people had come through similar feelings intact: it felt as though I was the first person ever to suffer in this particular way. The shock of finding myself unable to function was combined with the fear that this was *me*, now, that this was and was going to be my life, and down I spiralled.

So when young people I know and teach talk about 'my anxiety', for example, or when they explain that they find certain social situations unmanageable, I applaud them. They have done the research and taken control of the language. They understand that we all struggle, and they are acquiring the self-knowledge and the strategies which enable them to engage with the world on their terms. It is a huge step forward for us as individuals, for our societies and for ways of seeing and helping ourselves and each other. We are making real progress: if you are able to name (on your terms) what you are coping with, and make changes to help you cope, then you are part of that change.

5. But what *is* mental illness anyway?

Ready for a shock? OK, here goes: some of the most respected and knowledgeable people working in the field today, people who have helped many, many sufferers recover and heal, *do not like or use the term 'mental illness'*.

They prefer to talk about distress, and suffering, and well-being, and trauma – not illness. Because on the whole you cannot 'catch' mental problems; on the whole, as far as we can tell, they do not come from misfiring cells or systems, or unbalanced chemicals, or bacteria or viruses.

I say 'on the whole' because some conditions which present as extreme mental trauma *do* have a biological root – inflammation of the brain caused by auto-immune disease can cause psychosis; some forms of urinary tract infection cause an intense, delirious confusion.

But science has found nothing to indicate that most common kinds of mental distress are caused by anything 'wrong' with your body or brain.

God knows that mental suffering can cause the body and brain problems, from mild loss of appetite all the way to terrible damage. In periods when I have been miserable, I have lost weight, stopped exercising, stopped eating well and stopped sleeping properly. I become gaunt, exhausted, restless, incoherent, inarticulate: physically ill.

We know that recurrent depressions, including those you get with bipolar, are associated with increased chances of dementia – thanks to damage caused by high levels of cortisol in the brain of the depressed, it is thought. (Yeah, I know: ain't life grand? When I learned of this, I was struggling through the winter blues. And now I had dementia to look forward to. Thanks a *bunch*.)

Compared to many sufferers, my winter miseries are at the shallow end, but being in that physical state surely causes more mental suffering, which causes more physical symptoms. Anyone who has ever had an eating disorder can tell you about the tortures such a vicious cycle can inflict.

But the point is – we have *not* found a causal imbalance of chemicals, or a definitive genetic link between the body and mind. We suspect there are biological elements to some conditions – bipolar and depression seem to run in families, for example – but despite large-scale spending and research we have found no proof, no 'biomarkers'.

While some clinicians insist that if you are mentally suffering, then you should be understood and treated as mentally ill, others point to the fact that in mental health, suffering is not caused by 'disease': suffering, in this strange land of the mind that we are travelling through, does not come from physical things – or not as far as we know at the moment.

We can hope that neurobiologists and medical researchers find biomarkers and genetic and physical causes for as many mental conditions as possible, as soon as possible, and medical ways to treat them too, but until they do (and it is possible there are no biomarkers, no significant genetic or physiological causes) this country of ours will continue to be ruled by three main forces:

- environment and events – what has happened to you in your life, and what is happening now
- language – how you understand what is happening to you, how you think and speak of it (and how those around you do), and
- actions – what you (and those close to you) do about it.

And the good news is, although you cannot change whatever may have happened in the past, how you understood it or what you did, *you can and you must take control of all the rest now, and from now on.*

Time for a story, a very famous story, about how environment, language and action conspired to kill – and how things might have been different.

Imagine you are a sensitive young person, raised in privilege, from an extremely wealthy home. You have powerful and successful parents. You win a place at one of the best universities in Europe, where you do well. Then, in the middle of your course, you get terrible news from home: your father has died. Shortly after the funeral, your mother marries your father's brother, your uncle, who is an asshole, whom you hate.

You fall out very badly with your mum. You start to suffer a manic breakdown: you find yourself ranting and raving and talking to yourself. You suffer hallucinations and start hearing voices, believing a messenger from the spirit world wants you to kill your uncle, for the crime of murdering your dad.

Your mum's new husband, your asshole uncle, bullies you and instructs one of his mates to spy on you. You have a fight with this mate and end up killing him and stashing his corpse in a cupboard. As if that were not bad enough, your girlfriend, this dead guy's daughter, commits suicide. And now you get the strong feeling that your girlfriend's brother, in league with your uncle, is planning to kill you.

Luckily, your family is loaded. Needing help, you go private, skip the waiting lists and immediately get a long appointment with the psychiatrist, who is highly trained and a brilliant clinician.

She asks you a lot of questions about your life before all this happened. You talk about periods of low mood, which are common among young people and students, and then your feelings since your father died.

The psychiatrist listens and takes careful notes. Eventually, she says you appear to have a traumatic stress disorder brought about by your recent life events. She tells you that you are suffering from psychosis (the delusions which make you think you can see spirits) and auditory hallucinations (the voices you have been hearing), which could be the grounds for a schizophrenia diagnosis.

She says you have shown signs of a tendency to depression, often associated with winter: you come from a country in the north of Europe where rates of Seasonal Affective Disorder and suicide are high. You are obviously a sensitive, creative and highly intelligent person, she says.

Going on what you have told her, she says, she could diagnose you with a depressive disorder, cyclothymia, PTSD, SAD, psychosis, schizophrenia, bipolar, or all of the above, but she worries that you may not find this helpful. Instead, if you agree, she thinks it would be useful to apply a contemporary diagnosis, now extremely popular across Europe, which embraces all your symptoms.

You say that sounds sensible.

She gives you your diagnosis: melancholy.

She explains that although there is no cure, the symptoms of melancholy can be treated, and that by changing your routine and adopting certain healthy behaviours, you can and will make a recovery. If you are careful and committed to healing, she says, she is 100 per cent confident that you can and will live a full, long (unless you are run over by a bus) and happy life, with your melancholy under control.

You say that sounds good.

She books you a series of twenty appointments with a psychotherapist, starting in a couple of days' time, who specialises in trauma therapies. She gives you a book, *Brain Changer* by Felice Jacka, on how to change your diet. She recommends you engage a personal trainer to get you fit (it really helps that your family is rolling in cash). She suggests you contact your university and get mitigating circumstances, allowing you to take some time away from your course, and return when you are better. She says she will provide a full doctor's note, of course.

The psychiatrist now suggests that it might be a good idea to go to a retreat: she knows just the place, it has really nice gardens, it's by the sea, the food is terrific, they offer fabulous courses in gardening, painting, sculpture and creative writing. There was a good piece about it in *The Financial Times*, she says, and she shows you the article. The place looks great: the rooms are deluxe, en suite, of course, and the beds are massive.

You say you are definitely up for it.

And now she says you should think about taking up new activities: evidence shows this can have a great effect on people with melancholy. What do you enjoy?

You say you like fencing and shooting and reading and debating.

She says that's a good start, but how about something new: scuba diving, maybe? Skydiving? Have you thought of getting a pilot's licence? How about a hot-air balloon pilot's licence? She says doing yoga has been shown to be very helpful.

You say you like the sound of all of that.

Now she recommends you do some reading – you really like reading – about how your attitude and your thinking can change your situation, to the point of changing your fitness, your well-being and even your life expectancy. She recommends *The Expectation Effect* by David Robson. You decide to give it a go.

Finally, she explains that your melancholy will get dramatically worse if you do not rest and sleep and remove yourself from stressful situations. She strongly recommends that you get your best mate, H, who has come home from university to support you, to drive you to the retreat now – she will call ahead and make your reservation – and she gives you two pills, which she says are antipsychotics, also used as mood stabilisers.

'Take one this evening,' she says, 'and one tomorrow – the medication will help you sleep and stop you seeing ghosts and hearing voices.'

'OK,' you say.

She suggests you avoid your family completely, at least until you have done the retreat – she doesn't recommend any contact with them, at all, until you are feeling a lot stronger. They are obviously really triggering for you, she says, and she's talked to H, who agrees with her. She strongly recommends you stay off your phone – you have been posting a lot of mad stuff on social media recently, in your distress, and hanging out on a bunch of really nasty sites, including chat rooms where you have been debating the merits of suicide with other sufferers of melancholy.

'It might be a good idea to let H look after your phone for a couple of weeks,' she says, 'At least while you are on retreat?'

You agree.

She makes another appointment for you in two weeks' time, and gives you the number of her direct line: if you need to speak with her at any point, day or night, she says you should get the staff at the retreat to call her for you.

You are feeling so much better as you shake hands and thank her very much. You are massively relieved to have a diagnosis and a treatment plan. You are really looking forward to the retreat – especially being by the sea. You love sea swimming. You leave the appointment feeling like a new person, about a thousand times better than when you went in.

Unfortunately, just before you get into H's car to go to the retreat, you check your phone one last time. There is a message from your uncle inviting you to a fencing match with your girlfriend's brother, whose dead dad you hid in the cupboard. Your mum would also like to see you there, your uncle says. H says this sounds like a terrible idea and urges you to ignore it. But you reckon you can kick anyone's ass, sword-wise, definitely this twat who wants to fight you. You tell H not to worry; you've got this . . .

Soon after *Hamlet* was written and first performed, Robert Burton was writing his masterpiece, *The Anatomy of Melancholy*, which was published in 1621, and rapidly republished with many revisions and expansions. In four hundred years it has never been out of print. Rather like *Your Journey, Your Way*, the book is a compilation of case studies, but it is also much more – a work of dazzling non-fiction containing philosophy, theory, storytelling, wit, speculation, suggestion and, subtly, autobiography (one can only aspire). Its full title describes it: *The Anatomy of Melancholy, What it is: With all the Kinds, Causes, Symptomes, Prognostickes, and Several Cures of it. In Three Maine Partitions with their several Sections, Members, and Subsections. Philosophically, Medicinally, Historically, Opened and Cut Up.*

Though wonderfully rich and enjoyable, it is not light reading: it was last republished in 2001 and it runs to over 1,400 pages. (For a short cut, I recommend *A User's Guide to Melancholy* by Mary Ann Lund.) It is useful to consider, when thinking about how we suffer now, and how we understand suffering, that Hamlet is the classic Melancholy Man of the time.

In those days, it was thought our bodies contained balances and imbalances of the 'humours' – black bile, yellow bile, phlegm and blood – which made us feel and act in certain ways, depending also on the influence of the planets, and God. This may seem loopy now, but in four hundred years' time, many of the ways we currently understand and treat mental suffering will surely seem batty, too. It is worth remembering that we are only just beginning to get to grips with suffering, and that all our treatments are fairly recent works-in-progress.

Hamlet is also a modern man, for his time, inclined to believe more in science and reason than in ghosts and violent old traditions of vengeance and damnation. For Hamlet, going mad – or suffering acute mental distress, as we might now put it – can mean all kinds of things. It might mean that he was born damned, predestined to bring about his own tragedy. (If you have had depression, you will know that feeling: beating myself up in the midst of that darkness, I have often felt that the wreckage of my life, as it feels to me then, is entirely my own fault, and due to my bad character and selfish actions. Shame and guilt can be killers, especially when combined with breakdown.)

Hamlet also understands that seeming mad – or suffering a mental health crisis – can be very useful. One of my father's girlfriends, a photographer and picture editor, told me how she had survived exploring the wild bits of New York in the 1980s while working on a book about Lou Reed and the Velvet Underground – as an outsider, a woman, and someone of small stature and not physically strong – by pretending to be crazy when she felt threatened on the subway and in the rougher parts of the city. In the same way, many people who suffer now find forms of what Hamlet calls 'madness' a useful refuge from the pressures of life. 'I can't go to that (gig or drink or event) because of my blues,' I have often thought. And when I am in a cheerful mood and someone tells me about some bastard who has been hassling them, I sometimes say, 'Would you like me to sort him out? I have mental health, so I can do him over and be out in twenty-eight days.' It's silly and irresponsible, of course, but sometimes when you see one of my kind in a manic phase, ranting on a street corner in filthy rags, you might consider that this may be therapeutic behaviour for that person – it is healthy to let it all out, to express yourself, to communicate, howsoever wildly – and also that their scared and lonely selves may find this a rare safe place: half living but also half performing the role of the lunatic, the fool, someone mad and unsettling, someone worth going around, and in that way, defended.

Teaching at a university in Liverpool, I worked with many students who were having hard times. 'Anxiety' was just becoming a popular concept (we definitely didn't use the word at the University of York in the early nineties). I will never forget a message from one student who said they were on their way to our seminar when their anxiety got the better of them, just as they were entering the building where our department was, and they had decided to go home. I thought about it a lot. On one hand, the student had won a great battle and made a great decision: they had got out of bed feeling dreadful, but still got ready, left the house and gone into the university, and when it felt like it was all too much, they had made the wise choice to go home.

On the other hand, part of me felt that if they had just made it up the stairs to the seminar, not only would they have managed just fine, but the success of having pulled that off, the victory of going to class when feeling anxious, would have been a really good blow struck against their anxiety – proof that they had beaten it, at least for that day, and a reason to believe they could beat it again tomorrow.

I worried that they might have felt worse, returning to their accommodation having missed the seminar, than if they had not tried to go at all.

We all know that suffering can be a vicious cycle. The first time I met any kind of mental suffering was in my second year at university: I know now it was depression, but then it just felt like going mad with unhappiness.

Wonderfully, the student, through their own magnificent strength and determination, responded to the belief that my colleagues and their peers and I all had in them, overcame their anxiety, and triumphed. (They made a lot of good judgements which must have felt terrifying at the time, like going all the way to university and turning around before they reached the seminar.) We watched them perform at an open mic showcase at the end of the three-year course, and a lot of us cried. Not only had they beaten anxiety and depression, they had proved they could write and perform for an audience. They could speak in public; they could hold and move and entertain a rowdy audience. It was sublime to witness.

Compared to their courage, Hamlet's decision to accept the challenge of a possibly lethal sword fight looks brave, sure – but nowhere near as mighty. However, Hamlet also does the same thing they did when they decided to take their anxiety home, rather than to the seminar. Apologising to Laertes for killing his father, and fighting Laertes in his poor sister Ophelia's grave, Hamlet says:

> Was't Hamlet wronged Laertes? Never Hamlet:
> If Hamlet from himself be ta'en away,
> And when he's not himself does wrong Laertes,
> Then Hamlet does it not. Hamlet denies it.
> Who does it, then? His madness.

The reason I have brought that wonderful student and Hamlet into this chapter is language.

For me at university, the best terms for what I was going through were 'mad with unhappiness/depression'.

For our student it was 'anxiety'.

For Hamlet, 'madness'.

For his society, 'melancholy'.

And for me, for our student and for Hamlet, the thing behind the words, the feelings we use the words to describe – madness, melancholy or anxiety – could be real entities, our shadows, our doppelgängers stalking us, telling us that it is they who are real, that it is they who determine what we are and what will become of us. It is not true. But to defeat them we must own them, their names and their powers, so that once we have fought them we might befriend them.

How do we make our enemy our friend? I feel that a whole range of mental distress, which touches hundreds of millions, if not billions of people, encompassing all kinds of conditions, from insomnia to psychosis, via depression and eating disorders, and including moments of intense mental experience, like grief or love, could all be helpfully thought of as forms of madness. Madness is an ordinary part of human life. It's in all of us. It is not necessarily even a bad or scary thing. Think how we might describe a hilarious incident or a brilliant party: 'It was mad!'

All over Britain it is common to hear something or someone described as 'Mental!' Often it is not even a negative or critical term: it's more descriptive, and it can be affectionate, like 'wild' or 'crazy', as in this conversation I had in Llantwit Major when I asked a barman about a tennis match at Wimbledon.

'Did you see the men's final? How was it?'

'Oh, it was a really good first set but then he went mental and that was the end of it.'

When I was growing up in Wales with my brother, perhaps because our mother has always been very free in speaking her mind, we used to hear words and phrases like: loopy, bonkers, crazy, lunatic, fruitcake, maniac, crazy as a loon, loony, loony bin, barking, bats, mad as a snake, bananas, not all there, et cetera, all the time.

Mum would frequently and laughingly tell us we were 'complete maniacs' who were 'mad as snakes'. One of our neighbours, a tremendous lady known as Betty Cwmffrwdd, once called me out, when I was quite young, on using the phrase 'the loony bin' to describe our local mental hospital.

'Who taught you to say that?' she demanded.

'Mummy says it!'

'Well, will she call it that when she's in there?' Betty asked.

I remember thinking for a moment before I answered.

'Yes, she will,' I said.

I remember Betty rolling her eyes and suppressing a grin, but there is a really important point here. The English word 'mad' comes from the Old English, from the Germanic, *gemad* meaning 'changed' or 'changed for the worse'.

This is a simple and accurate term for all kinds of distress in which you or your life feel changed for the worse. I find it healthy and helpful to think of the ways I have suffered, and all the myriad other ways in which so many of us suffer, as normal, ordinary and common variations of 'changed for the worse'.

Considering that we begin our existence in a lovely warm womb, and progress through being cradled and fed to growing up, going to school, trying to get and keep jobs and money, surviving, thriving, fighting for or failing to find security and happiness, until we age and head towards all the trials that age can bring, including challenges to our health, finances and well-being, and death, human life could accurately be considered a condition of *gemad* – change, perhaps change for the worse. It is indeed a mad life, and the world is surely very mad a lot of the time.

*

In mythology, when you meet a dragon, you need to know its name. Give your pain or fear or threat a name, and you have taken a vital step towards confronting it. As we have seen, diagnosis in mental health produces a broad category name for a specific individual condition. Someone else has named your dragon for you, but they don't know it as well as you do, or have to live with it inside them. And it attracts other dragons, including one of the worst, most damaging and terrifying: stigma.

Stigma is an absolute bastard of a dragon: I was posting blithely on social media about the importance, as I saw it, of coming out about mental health and being honest about our situations, our sufferings and our conditions. A correspondent messaged me to say he would not advise anyone in his workplace to come out with a mental health condition. They would be stigmatised instantly, he said.

Privilege is the reason I am able to own my own variety of madness. My line managers at the University of Manchester are entirely understanding, and (expertly) ever supportive. My other jobs, books, journalism and broadcasting, allow me huge freedom and latitude: I do not have to do work that does not interest me; I can take siestas; I work at home or from anywhere I like; I am often cash poor but in freedom and self-determination I am fundamentally rich. So it is relatively easy for me to tell myself and others that my dragon does not own me. Handily, that often means standing on a stage and announcing that I have been as crazy as a cricket, as mad

YOUR JOURNEY, YOUR WAY

as a snake, a loony, a nutter, a mentalist, which is a form of talking therapy for me, paying in attention, connectedness, meaning, a sense of identity which gives me validation, and actual cash. This is exactly what Robert Burton did in his *Anatomy of Melancholy*: he said he wrote about melancholy 'by being busy to avoid melancholy'. I find talking about my breakdown is a great therapy for me. Ahmed Hankir is a practising psychiatrist and the performer of a show, 'The Wounded Healer', about breakdown and healing. His public role, he says, is one of the ways he keeps his bipolar in lifelong remission.

Stigma has taken some hits, thanks to the pandemic. We talk more and more frankly about our mental health. There is a wider public acknowledgement that we are all capable of mental suffering. But stigma is still a dragon, and you do not want language to become one of its claws. You need language on your side.

By far the most dangerous aspect of stigma does not come from outside you – we're not worrying about people pointing at us in the street and jeering at us for being depressed or anxious or whatever. No, the issue here is the stigma that comes from within.

If you spend time telling yourself, 'I have anxiety / I am depressed / I have a disorder,' it is very difficult to find ease or happiness. The 'inner critic' is bullying you. Screw that. When those thoughts come, I might think, 'What the hell?! So now I'm going to stigmatise *myself*? Oh please . . .' God knows I've done it often enough.

The key point here is this. You are much bigger, much

stronger and much more significant than any words used to describe your condition, be they medical, 'scientific' or popular terms you hear in the pub or online. Make sure you own your language, and do not be frightened, ever, by anyone else's. (Remember Rule 2: You call it what you want!)

Because, after all:

Rule 5: Madness is in all of us, and the world is surely mad.*

We are now ready for the next chapter, and some of the best news this book contains.

Whatever has happened to you, whatever you have done, however you feel, whatever you have been told, psychology and the most successful treatments we have so far discovered have an amazing piece of news for you:

You are normal.

Seriously. *Your behaviours and your feelings are an entirely normal, understandable and common reaction to the pressures you have been under.*

---

* Read as much of the *Daily Mail* online as you can in ten minutes. I rest my case.

6. The cutting edge: A message of lifesaving hope (from Finland)

After I had been sectioned and treated (two doses of quetiapine, a couple of weeks in a psychiatric ward, staged return to the community, and a prescription for aripiprazole, which I took for a couple more weeks before tapering myself off and lying about it) and I had reached a kind of fragile recovery period, still shaky, but working again, I found myself in my flat one dark winter evening, talking to Yasmin Ishaq on the phone.

Yasmin has been a social worker for thirty-five years, a psychotherapist for ten years, and worked as an AMHP (Approved Mental Health Professional) for fifteen years. AMHPs have a particular role in making out the order to detain under the Mental Health Act when someone is sectioned. It's not a doctor who sends you to hospital when you do not want to go – it's an AMHP.

Yasmin is an extraordinary woman, astonishingly gentle and respectful, and since 2014, when she trained as an Open Dialogue practitioner in the UK and Finland, she has been part of the spread of this remarkable treatment across the UK. She led the first trial of Open Dialogue in England, in Kent.

I was fascinated by Open Dialogue, because I was

desperately looking for a way out of the rather terrifying place I found myself.

I did not want to take the aripiprazole, or anything else (I was terrified of the very many side effects, and the way it seemed to numb me, and affect my work).

I did not want to go mad again.

I did not want to tell my partner that I was determined to come off aripiprazole, for fear she would dump me and I would lose much of my time with and access to our son, and her.

But however much I googled bipolar and cyclothymia, however much I read, I was really struggling to find a way out of what felt like a binary trap: pills or madness.

And then I found Open Dialogue.

It was not the only answer I came across – thanks to my generous and wealthy father I was able to afford more than ten weeks of therapy, during which I did Eye Movement Desensitisation and Reprocessing, which was a life-changer (we shall come back to EMDR) – but it looked and felt like a breakthrough.

Here was a minimal medication treatment, developed in Finland, that reported stunning results. Stunning really is the word. Over 70 per cent success rate for recovery / return to work or study, and for the most severe conditions, too – psychosis and voice hearing – versus 9 per cent success rate for the UK's treatment-as-usual programmes, which rely on medication.

But there were a number of problems, which you or

any sufferer you know will probably face too, at least for some years after this book is published.

- There were very few Open Dialogue programmes running in the UK.
- Those which were taking on patients tended to be in trial areas.
- To get on those trials, you had to live in a certain postcode (in Kent, in this case).
- Even if you happened to live in Kent, and met the criteria for enrolment, you were not guaranteed a place – you would also have to be very lucky, to be picked.

We were heading towards the first pandemic lockdown, so although Yasmin was happy to recommend me to some of her patients, which would have allowed me to speak with them and begin to really understand Open Dialogue from a sufferer's point of view, I couldn't go to Kent to meet them.

Conclusion: Open Dialogue was closed to me, as it may well be closed to you.

BUT, Yasmin was extremely generous with her time, and she spent ages with me on the phone, as I smoked out of the window of my bedroom and scribbled down what she said in my notebook, balanced on my window sill.

What she told me changed my life, and I would like you to know about it, because the four years I have so far spent researching mental health treatments have convinced me of two things, above all.

1. In fifty or a hundred years' time, we will not treat people who are suffering in anything like the way we do now.
2. The techniques Open Dialogue uses will be a large part of the answer.

I asked her: Yasmin, if I came to you and said I was bipolar, that two psychiatrists and everything I have read on the web confirm I am bipolar, what would you say?

She said: Well, I wouldn't take it away from you; I'd never take a diagnosis away from someone if they found it helpful, but I would say that I don't find it helpful. I would say, for the purposes of this treatment, let's just leave it to one side for now. I am much more interested in what has happened to you, in your life and family circumstances, in what you have been going through and in what you are feeling now. I would start there.

Fine, I said. I can do that. But supposing I came to you, as mad as a hatter, and told you that I am working with the world's intelligence agencies on a great secret global movement to bring about world peace and a revolution in consciousness, that I am in contact with aliens, and that I am engaged to be married to Kylie Minogue?

This was not a random or frivolous fantasy. When I was crazy (or 'experiencing a psychotic episode, lacking insight, in a florid state, with flights of ideas and delusions') that is exactly what I believed. More than believed: I *knew* it was all true, knew it and saw it and felt it, as clearly and certainly as I can see my laptop screen now, and feel the keys under my fingers as I type. And I have to say, being engaged to Kylie was one of the best things about going nuts. What a lovely person she is.

Yasmin said: I would say, 'That is a perfectly normal, entirely understandable reaction to the situation you are in. It's a normal reaction to the pressure you are under.' That's the first thing we do: we normalise it.

This sounds simple, but in real terms, it is an enormous, momentous, world-changing point.

Do you have terrible insomnia? Do you have horrible, miserable, heart-crushing anxiety? That means you are *normal*. You are reacting to circumstances in your life or events in your life story, or both, in a normal, usual, common, human way.

Are you so depressed you wake up and wish you hadn't? Does the thought of leaving the house fill you with exhaustion and dread? That means you are normal. You are reacting to circumstances in your life or events in your life story, or both, in a normal, usual, common, human way.

Whether you have an eating disorder, psychosis, a borderline personality diagnosis, SAD, voice hearing, agoraphobia, anxiety, post-traumatic stress disorder, a schizophrenia diagnosis or any other kind of mental suffering, Open Dialogue has news for you: you are normal.

You are reacting to circumstances in your life or events in your life story, or both, in a normal, usual, common, human way.

Rule 6: You are normal, and likely not especially different to anyone else. You feel different because pressure, trauma, unhappiness, or something in your life or history, is making you feel and act in certain ways. Anyone in your position would feel and act the same way.

So this was obviously a massive moment for me, and I think about it a great deal. Yasmin was telling me, in effect, that there was nothing fundamentally 'wrong' with my brain. My brain and body react in certain ways to certain triggers: cannabis, lack of sleep, winter (can make me blue), summer (can make me a bit high) and the pressures of life events, and my reactions to them (lying, cheating, drinking too much, running to keep up with myself, et cetera) can and will drive me crazy, if I don't deal with them. But there is no chemical imbalance in my brain, no fundamental flaw. I can go mad, and I can definitely, easily drive myself mad, but the fundamental fact is *I am not mad* – or at least, no more mad than anyone else. And the same is true for you, and for everyone you love and care about.

At least, that is what Open Dialogue practitioners believe. And the British Psychological Society believes the same thing. Psychologists do not ask 'What is wrong with you?' but rather, 'What has happened to you?'

Psychiatrists might like to take the same approach, and many do, but they lack the time (on the NHS): they have to deal with what is in front of them, and quickly, under immense pressure, so they tend to deal with your symptoms, rather than what is causing them. This normally means medication.

Open Dialogue makes no criticism of psychiatry, and many psychologists don't either – although it has to be said, many other psychologists *do* criticise psychiatry, and fiercely. But psychiatrists have a clinician's desire and a legal duty to do whatever they can to make sure you do not, in your distress, harm yourself or anyone else.

Your psychiatrist wants to improve your life, and fast. If they fail – if you leave a psychiatrist's appointment and hurt yourself or someone else – as well as feeling upset and perhaps responsible, your psychiatrist is liable to find themselves in the Coroner's Court, answering questions at an inquest. In their shoes, I would be pretty quick to prescribe medication, too. I believe I would have done what my psychiatrists did when they tried to treat me: I think I would have prescribed medication, too. And I hope I would have said, when pushed, which one of them did when I pushed him, 'Well, it's your life – I can't make you take it. If you don't want to take it, don't.'

When I was in the midst of psychotic delusions (sorry, Kylie) the thing that really helped me was those two doses of quetiapine. They made me feel ghastly, but they worked.

If someone I loved very much and worried about very much was in the same place, I would want them to have antipsychotic medication too, and fast. The loxapine

I was given by the French trauma specialist, and the instruction, 'Take one if you feel you are going high, or not getting enough sleep,' has been incredibly helpful, on the two or three occasions I have taken it.

Anyway, when Yasmin is doing Open Dialogue, she has a clinician, a doctor or a psychiatrist who is qualified to prescribe medication, in the room with her. If the sufferer ('service user' is the technical, NHS-approved term; personally I prefer 'sufferer' or 'patient') needs medication, they get it.

But the fundamental practice of Open Dialogue is that patients should be prescribed minimal doses of medication, only when absolutely necessary, and that they should take it for the minimum possible time.

(This is only a personal opinion, but my own strong feeling is that this principle should be applied to all kinds of mental health medication in all situations. I would bet anything that it will come to be standard practice in the future – but it definitely is not standard practice now.)

We will come back to medication, but for now, and to prepare for that section:

Rule 7: Medication can be a lifesaver, but most psychiatric medication can only treat symptoms, not causes.

7. Techniques you and your support network can take from Open Dialogue, even if you cannot access it

So how does Open Dialogue work? The treatment is based on seven principles. They are:

1. immediate help
2. social network perspective
3. flexibility and mobility
4. responsibility
5. psychological continuity
6. tolerance of uncertainty
7. dialogue (and polyphony).

Supposing I have had a breakdown, and believe I am working with spies and aliens and engaged to you-know-who, due to a conversation I have been having with the television (which is what happened), this is what Open Dialogue means.

1. Immediate help

I get an appointment very quickly. On Day 1 I am getting out my best suit and polishing my smart shoes and informing my radio, which I believe is listening to me, that the head of MI6 better be there in church tomorrow when I walk down the aisle with a celebrated Australian superstar or else my friend ET is going to turn up in his flying saucer and zap Vauxhall Cross (MI6 HQ) with a big laser, and therefore am clearly bonkers (lacking insight and suffering delusions, and making my partner and friends believe I may harm myself or others). Open Dialogue aims to start my treatment on that day, Day 1 – or on Day 2, or as soon as possible.

Important to note: just because it does not happen quickly does not stop it working. I interviewed the relative of a sufferer who had been on psychiatric wards several times and seemed to be hurtling towards suicide when they found themselves in Open Dialogue treatment. It saved and changed their life.

2. Social network perspective

It is not just me in the treatment room. Sitting side by side with me are my partner, my friends Doug and Ellie (two dear friends and neighbours who were amazing when I had the breakdown, and really helped to look after me, my partner and our child), perhaps my mum, or someone else from my social network who is close to me, an Open Dialogue practitioner (like Yasmin Ishaq), a peer supporter (this could be me, now: someone who has been through a breakdown and therefore understands how frightened, lonely, confused and perhaps defensive the sufferer is feeling), a clinician (a doctor or psychiatrist) and perhaps a second member of Yasmin's Open Dialogue team. The point is, Open Dialogue is not just treating me. It's also treating my partner, our friends and my mother, in this case.

This is the opposite of your experience now, assuming you have a breakdown: it will either be just you in the room, facing the psychiatrist – and perhaps an assistant, who may be a student medic (such was my experience, twice), and possibly your partner or someone close to you. Whoever else is there, as the sufferer you are left in no doubt that this is all about you, about whatever is wrong with you, that you are in the frame, and that the problem here is what is going on in your brain: everyone else's brain is fine. They are all upset and worried, and that's because of you. One of the great breakthroughs of Open Dialogue is that it treats the network, not just the individual.

3. Flexibility and mobility

Yasmin says a lot of the secret of Open Dialogue is down to diaries and scheduling. This first appointment is not a one-off. It may need to be the first of several.

Assuming I was bonkers on Day 1, and the first meeting took place on Day 2, the second may need to take place on Day 3, which will probably mean everyone has to juggle their schedules and adjust their diaries. It may have to take place in a different venue from the first – in my flat, for example, or in my partner's living room – but the point is, everyone involved has to do their utmost to make sure that second meeting, and the third and the fourth, as required, really do happen when they need to happen.

4. Responsibility

This is where it starts to become really interesting. Following Yasmin's leadership (using her as an example, in this case) everyone is invited to share how they are feeling now. Not about how they feel about the prospect of me marrying you-know-who, with James Bond and M and Q standing in the congregation: how they are feeling in themselves, today, now. So:

My partner says she has been having a stressful time, but she is relieved to be here.

Doug and Ellie agree, and say they have been worried about her and me and our boy.

I say I am a bit frustrated, because there is nothing wrong with me and I need to get ready for my wedding.

My mum says she is just so relieved that I am safe, now, here, and that she feels very grateful and lucky that we have this appointment, and admits she has been worrying a lot, and so is rather tired.

Yasmin says she is in a good place, and very happy everyone could make it here today, and so she is also feeling optimistic, because we seem to her a good, strong, wide network.

The doctor says she's had a busy day, so she's been a bit stressed, but she finds these sessions very valuable, and she's glad to feel the positive energy and hope in the room.

The peer supporter says he is concerned for me, because he knows what it is like, and he's worried that I don't seem to have slept much in the last few days, if at all.

The assistant practitioner says he feels concern for the worry we have all been going through, as a network, but like Yasmin, is optimistic, because we are obviously a caring and supportive group.

The point is, without explicitly being told to do it, everyone is taking responsibility for their own feelings. It's not about me, the sufferer, and whatever I have or have not done. It's about all of us. We are sitting side by side, and working side by side, already. Yasmin and her team have begun to normalise a chaotic and scary situation. We have all formed a team, already, a team that will only get stronger as we go further – and we have had our first lesson. We are taking responsibility for how we all feel. Furthermore, Yasmin and the doctor, with help from the peer supporter and the assistant practitioner, are taking clinical responsibility for all of us. We cannot help but relax a bit. We are in wonderful hands.

The next thing that happens is we all share our fears. So:

My partner says she knows I need real help, she thinks I need to go to hospital, and she's scared I might talk my way out of it.

I say there is nothing wrong with me, and I am scared of being sectioned and made to take medication I believe I really don't need.

My mother says she is scared that if I do get sectioned I'll be frightened and perhaps over-medicated (she's heard some bad things about what can happen in hospital).

Doug says he is worried for me, because he knows how lonely and sleepless I have been, and he wants me to get a rest, and that would be the best thing for my partner, too: it's been a frantic time for her, and she needs a break.

The doctor says she worries that I am overtired, and that my partner is too, and that she feels a really strong responsibility to make sure I get some rest, at the very least.

Ellie says she is worried about my partner, who has been trying so hard, and my mum, who has come a long way to be here, and about me, because I really do need a rest.

My peer supporter says he knows how it feels to not want to go to hospital or take medication when you feel the way I do, and that if he was in my shoes, he'd want to have a guarantee he was not going to be sectioned, and was not going to have to take medication.

Yasmin and her assistant use their hands and touch their chests or stomachs when they talk about how they feel. They say they both feel a bit tense, in their stomachs, because of all the worry in the room, but they also feel very moved by all the love and care and concern in the room. They invite us all to do the same thing. To take a minute to think about how we are feeling, and where in the body we are feeling it, and whether tension and stress have gone down since the session started.

Also, their mode of speaking is very humble, very respectful. Although they are the experts in the treatment, they do not act or speak as though they are in charge, or have any kind of authority. So:

Yasmin and her assistant encourage the doctor to share more of her fears about responsibility for me.

And then my peer supporter.

And then me.

Yasmin agrees with me, that the idea of being forced to go anywhere or take anything would be really frightening, if she was in my shoes.

And then we go round again. And again.

Doug makes a joke. My partner and my mother (who have not always got on, which has been a part of the stress leading to my breakdown, in this imaginary example) both laugh. They both love Ellie and Doug, and they bond over that, and the same worries about me they have all been sharing.

Yasmin makes the point that the things I have been doing and saying and believing are not a sign that I have a defective brain or that there is anything deeply wrong with me: in effect, my delusions are a kind of language I am using to describe and create an alternative reality; a reality I can bear. My life circumstances – not sleeping, fighting with my partner, taking drink and drugs, risk-taking behaviour, fear that people think I am 'bipolar', et cetera have made my reality unbearable. That is all this is: a really normal, actually quite sensible reaction to the pressure and unhappiness of my situation.

My mum and my partner and Doug and Ellie start to show signs of real relief. Their dear son/friend/partner is behaving in a common way, which Yasmin and her team and the doctor do not find alarming or scary at all. Yasmin says she's worked with a lot of people in situations like mine and none of them are now banged up on a locked ward or struggling with the side effects of powerful medication. They are fine. They are healing. Most of them are back at work, or heading that way. Their friendships and relationships within their networks were actually strengthened by going through breakdown and healing together. And with such a strong network as this, she is quite sure that's what is going to happen to us.

The peer supporter tells the brief story of his own breakdown. He was experiencing a whole lot of hassle from GCHQ and MI5 but it turned out he just really needed a proper rest, and a lot of perspective, and a change of job, and a better diet, and therapy – he had a lot of therapy, because it turned out he was being driven crazy by rampaging perfectionism, which he and his therapist traced back to childhood trauma. Now he looks back on it, it was actually one of the best things that ever happened to him, because it helped him change his life in healthy ways.

And so we go round again.

Each time we go round, more stress and fear and pressure leave us. As our guards drop, our emotions come out, more humour and love and kindness and trust. Crying, at one point, we start telling each other how much we love each other, and how worried we have been.

We never feel a sense of time pressure while we are working together. Yasmin and her team emphasise that we can take as long as we like, to share and to listen and to feel.

Meanwhile, the strangest thing is happening to me. When I came in, I was in defensive, threat-response, fight-or-flight mode. I assumed they were all going to gang up on me and tell me I was crazy and section me and pill me up. Instead, I'm hearing I'm normal, or at least reacting in normal ways. We all seem to be on the same side. I am finding it easy to trust Yasmin and her assistant. And the peer supporter has really got my back, and even the doctor seems on my side. And I'm beginning to see how I can help my dear friends and my mum, and even my partner. In the back of my mind I am beginning to see a trade here: if they don't make me go to hospital, I could agree to take one pill. Christ, I'm a nineties kid! I can take double anything Withnail can . . . how much harm could one or two do?

5. Psychological continuity

What we are not going to do, with this rather wonderful thing we have all made, this place of listening, and courage, and faith in each other, is let it drop. Perhaps not everyone in the network can make the next meeting – but Yasmin can, my peer supporter can, Yasmin's assistant can, the doctor can (barring emergencies), and Doug can. So we keep the network going. Although my partner can't make it, because she has our child to look after, and she's desperate not to have to miss too many more classes (she's a teacher, and it's coming up to exam time), Doug and Yasmin will speak to her before the next session and find out how she is, what she would have liked to say and share in the session, and any points she would like to make. The whole strength of the programme is that I as the sufferer feel safe and understood, or at least as understood and listened to as possible.

Three twenty-minute appointments across three months with two different psychiatrists with different (and changing) assistants in the room, which was my experience of treatment-as-usual, this is *not*.

In that situation, in the situation of most people going to see most doctors and psychiatrists, the experience of the sufferer depends entirely on the skill of the clinician. That doctor or psychiatrist is either incredibly good at their job, being warm and attentive and thoughtful and respectful and empathetic and imaginative and effective, or they are not.

The two psychiatrists I met, one on the ward, and one a few weeks after I was released, may have been all those things, but it was hard to tell. They didn't really have time to listen to me. I didn't trust that they were thinking about me as an individual. And they both seemed to have made up their minds about me, from the notes on my case, before I walked into their rooms.

They told me what I was, what was wrong with me, and that I needed medication. They gave me to understand, above all, that they had power and expertise; I did not. It was only a personal experience, and not to be taken as a general criticism of psychiatry, but my experience of psychiatry made me feel lonely, misunderstood, suspicious, sceptical, unheard, unimportant – and also, because of my questions and doubts, psychiatry made me feel that I was, basically, rather annoying and difficult.

6. Tolerance of uncertainty

This is such a good one, I use it in my teaching when I am working with new writers and students. It means that rather than giving my students the impression that I know everything, or even very much, about how, say, the university is going to handle the pandemic and online teaching, or how strikes by lecturers will affect their teaching hours and their degrees/MAs, or how easy or hard it will be for them to break into publishing after the course (we work on creative non-fiction), or how the book they are working on will turn out, I say, look, I don't know. No one really knows. When it comes to things I can find out, I will try my best to find out what I can and I will definitely get back to you. And instead of finding it undermining that the 'authority figure' does not have all the answers, they find the honesty refreshing and even reassuring. In the context of Open Dialogue, it means that Yasmin says, 'I don't know for sure, but . . .' a lot.

So, for example, she might say, 'I don't know how long this session is going to take. I don't know what state Horatio will be in, a week from now. I don't know how many sessions we are going to need. I don't know how we will all be feeling tomorrow, or at the next session. I don't know exactly what you would call his condition. Do we need to call it anything except distress and exhaustion? I don't know how Horatio – and we all – are going to react to the Open Dialogue treatment. But what I can do is be open about my uncertainty, and sit with it. Rather than trying to hide it, or unloading it in the form of stress or pressure on anyone else, I am going to acknowledge it. And I am going to carry it and own it and accept that uncertainty is not just a part of life, but a huge part of the complicated world of well-being.'

By modelling this way of thinking and behaving, Yasmin encourages everyone in the group to admit, share and sit with their own uncertainties, and to acknowledge that uncertainty is normal, honest and healthy. So rather than conceal her own fears and uncertainties, as a conventional psychiatrist might when confronted with a complex and distressed patient, Yasmin is frank about them in front of everyone, including her peers and the team she leads. When we have worked together subsequently, I have seen that she always explains how she responds to significant developments and information: she will say, 'When you said [whatever it was] I could really feel how much it meant to you, and I felt [whatever she did] as I was listening to you. I feel it here . . .' Sometimes Yasmin will locate the feeling in her torso and describe it. The effect of such honesty and such painstaking acknowledgement and sharing is striking: if people sit with and express how they feel, and no one unloads their uncertainty (in the form of stress, anxiety, criticism or reproach, for example) on anyone else, then no one triggers a defensive or aggressive reaction in anyone else, and the group, the network, becomes a calmer, safer-feeling and ever-more effective place of change and development.

Again, this is the opposite approach from the one my psychiatrists took. They gave the impression that they knew what was wrong with me, and what that meant, and what sort of pills I should take. They had knowledge and insight; I did not. They had power; I did not. In truth, they were uncertain on which pills would be best for me. They gave me a choice of lithium, aripiprazole and sodium valproate. We do not know clearly how these pills work; we have hypotheses, to which individual clinicians do or do not subscribe; but we do know that the drugs have effects and side effects. When I asked my second psychiatrist how aripiprazole worked, he said, 'If you're up it brings you down, if you're down it brings you up!'

At the time I did not realise that the idea that there was a chemical imbalance in my brain was a widespread misconception, a debunked theory which psychiatry and neuroscience have disowned, but I knew I didn't understand how adding a chemical could both add to and subtract from that balance. The psychiatrists were right: I did not know the first thing about brain chemistry. But what would have been amazing, what would have really helped, would have been for one of them to say:

'Look, we don't really understand the brain. We know that these pills have certain beneficial effects in cases like yours. It would reassure us if you took them. We don't really know how they work, but statistically, we do know that people are less likely to have manic episodes if they take them. We feel worried for you and we are legally responsible for you. We can admit it: one of the reasons we are asking you to take them is because it will reassure us that you are less likely to do something which hurts someone. We don't want you to hurt yourself or anyone else, and we don't want to end up answering questions in a Coroner's Court, or under professional investigation, if you do. And we are just as concerned as you are that you should take the minimum dose for the minimum time. We are here to make sure that happens, and to help you taper down to the minimum or zero dosages as soon as safely possible. How does that sound?'

But because psychiatrists and doctors learn to carry themselves with a certain authority (which most of us enjoy, after all – you should see me showing off and yabbering on about writing), the last thing most of them do is admit to uncertainty. Who can blame them?

We, the sufferers and our families, put doctors and psychiatrists under huge psychological pressure to have the answer, to know what to do, to reassure us things are going to be OK – or, at least, better. So clinicians want to project competence, confidence and certainty, of course they do. The problem is, there is very little certainty in mental health. And being crazy or distressed does not make you blind or stupid. You can tell when someone is bluffing, even a little bit (I know I could), and if you are in a defensive, manic or paranoid state, you do not react well to that insight.

I have done many training and speaking sessions with psychiatrists, treatment teams and mental health pharmacists as a 'lived experience' adviser. Everything I have said here I have either learned from them or said to them. There have been no objections so far, and the psychiatrists I have worked with are notably keen to learn and adjust their practice based on all and any new information which strikes them as sensible and helpful.

I find it useful to remember this:

Rule 8: We suffer as individuals, but we are treated as categories. You are dealing with an overloaded, underfunded and creaky system. Insist on your treatment being as individual as possible.

The massive and obvious difference is that in Open Dialogue, we are treated as individuals and as a networked group of individuals. In standard practice, we are treated as a member of a very broad category or categories.

7. Dialogue (and polyphony)

You know you are doing a decent job, as a teacher, when your class, your seminar group (or your audience, if you're doing a talk about mental health at a literary festival, for example) are speaking, and you are not. Parenting is similar, as parents know: when the children are talking to each other, entertaining and (however comically or chaotically) informing and educating each other, you know you are doing well.

In the same way, Open Dialogue works by not privileging any voice above any other: polyphony means 'many voices'. Yasmin and her teams see themselves as facilitators, not authorities. They do not make any kind of big thing of their expertise or experience. Their aim is for the network to stand together, in a place of shared care and hope, and move together, bringing themselves and each other to a better place at the end of the session than they were at the beginning. The secret is simple: honest and respectful dialogue. The key is polyphony: many voices, all with equal status.

As it happens, findings in Finland, where Open Dialogue was invented, concern businesses, not health care. The Nordic model of flattened-hierarchy companies has been spreading throughout the region for decades: businesses have found that ditching vertical top-down structures of a boss at the top, with her subordinates below her, in charge of their subordinates below them, and so on, achieves startling results. Suppose I am making a radio programme in a flattened-hierarchy company and I run into problems – technical, legal, ethical, whatever. Conventionally, in a normal business or corporation, I take that problem to my boss: I 'refer up', as the BBC phrase has it. That was drummed into me. As long as you 'refer up' you are covered if it all goes belly-up. If your boss is also stuck on how to resolve it, they refer up to their boss, et cetera. In effect, in order to progress you pass stress, pressure and responsibility up the chain. If you want to progress – or if you are pressurised to progress – by making things work better, faster and cheaper, then you pass pressure, stress (and possibly cuts) down the chain. No wonder a lot of companies and institutions are tough places to work, with stressed bosses and pressurised employees.

But these Nordic flattened-hierarchy companies do not work this way. Rather than refer up, if I get stuck on my radio programme, I ask one of my colleagues. I explain the problem. We put our heads together, in dialogue. If we can't crack it, we ask another colleague, and if necessary another: we get a polyphony going. In the end, we come up with the best solution that we as a group can think of. I implement it. If it goes wrong, we know we tried: we all tried, and as a bonus we all understand the nature of the problem when it comes to making Plan B, because we are all already part of tackling it.

Statistics Finland, the state office for data collection and analysis, reports that relatively flat hierarchies lead employees to report high levels of direct communication, high levels of teamwork and significant levels of autonomy. The share of Finnish employees who feel they can influence important decisions at work is the highest on the Continent: 57 per cent, compared to the European average of 40 per cent.

Using the same principles, Yasmin Ishaq found that her Open Dialogue team reported higher levels of job satisfaction and well-being than workers in the conventional vertical hierarchy areas of the NHS. Staff turnover and days off sick in the Open Dialogue team were the lowest in the Kent and Medway NHS Foundation Trust.

Flattened hierarchy and dialogic working are not radical departures or strokes of innovative genius: their straightforward principles are in widespread practice throughout the Nordic countries, contributing to societies where workers and children consistently report the highest levels of happiness and lowest levels of stress in the world. Open Dialogue would seem to be a natural progression of what is effective in the workplace to what is effective in health treatment.

Open Dialogue is strikingly more effective than the treatment model you are likely to encounter. For the most severe afflictions – psychosis and voice hearing or schizophrenia – we currently have a (roughly) 9 per cent return to work/study rate in 2 to 5 years. The vast majority, if not all, of those people are on medication. Open Dialogue delivers a (roughly) 70 per cent return rate in the same period, and most of those people are on no medication or very little medication. The implications for sufferers, their families, their networks, their employers/employees and co-workers, and the implications for the NHS and the economy, are staggering. Yasmin's Kent trial found they needed one tenth of the bed-days of the treatment-as-usual model. Psychiatric acute care beds are incredibly expensive: representing a 90 per cent saving in this area, as well as the savings on medication, which is a fat slice of the NHS mental health budget. In 2020/21, the NHS spent £371 million on antidepressants and nearly £33 million on antipsychotics, according to analysis of NHS business data by the *Pharmaceutical Journal* and Wilmington Healthcare. Value for money is one of the reasons Open Dialogue is currently being carefully studied, trialled and rolled out in a growing selection of areas across the UK, Europe and the world.

Although this chapter has taken an imaginary example

of psychosis, or breakdown, it seems to me that this way of working together, treating the whole network, not just the sufferer, has tremendous possibilities for all kinds of mental distress. You may have heard the (slightly coarse) modern aphorism: *Before you decide you're clinically depressed, make sure you're not surrounded by assholes.*

I was surrounded by some of the wisest, kindest and most caring people I have ever come to know and love, but the pressure we were all under, due to my cracking up, was ferocious. It is well known among clinicians, approved mental-health professionals, home-based treatment teams and early intervention teams that the home and social environment of the sufferer is often a huge part of the problem.

(This is why I think psychiatric hospitals should be rebranded as retreats: just getting away for a couple of weeks, away from the worried faces of family and friends, and being in a quiet and calm ward, gave me a deep rest that I desperately needed. Just as important, it gave everyone else a break from me. Although I was very lucky with that ward, its staff and my group of fellow patients, one of my correspondents got in touch to say that when she was growing up in Liverpool it was quite common for women with heavy responsibilities, guiding their families through tough social and economic conditions, to go away 'for a rest' for a few days or weeks. Only years later did she realise that they had been short-stay patients in asylums. She said it was understood that they needed the break, and it helped.)

My point is: *The worst thing you can do for a sufferer (doubly so, if that person is you) is make them feel different or weird or alone.*

If you are one of the people who loves them, who is trying to help them, the worst thing for you is that feeling of responsibility and isolation. They are reacting to pressure in a normal human way. You are reacting to pressure on them and on you in a normal human way: this may be making you desperately worried, anxious or depressed; you may experience difficulty eating or sleeping. You may not have time or the ability to do the things you enjoy, the things that make you *you*. Being a carer, relative or partner to someone who is suffering can be worse than being the sufferer. In the case of my breakdown and my partner and friends, we are quite sure that it was a lot more fun for me, often, being mad, than it was for my partner who was trying to help me, and trying to raise our boy, and to keep her job, and to hold it all together. I have met many readers at events where I talk openly about mental health, often parents, and most often mothers, who feel they are in dire and desperately worrying situations, trying to get help for their adult children.

This is why treating the whole network and the sufferer as equally afflicted and equally in need of Open Dialogue is not some hippy Finnish philosophy. It is absolutely vital to the sufferer and their network that the well-being of everyone involved should be supported.

This is why groups who have taken part in Open Dialogue go all starry-eyed when they talk about that first ever session. For the first time, the carers, the family, the partner, the friends and the sufferer feel listened to and heard. For the first time, everyone has agency. For the first time, everyone has support. For the first time, everyone is in this together, and coming up with ways forward together. For the first time, the system does not seem insanely rushed and pressured. For the first time, caring and worried people are being asked how they feel, what they fear, what they need.

Now, we began this chapter with the sad fact that you are probably not going to be able to access Open Dialogue for a while, unless you are very lucky. But the principles and how they work are worth knowing. You never know how you might be able to apply them. The big thing for me, the thing that made me cry when I thought about it, was imagining how all of my loved ones' lives would have been different if we had had this sort of networked, peer-supported, dialogic treatment.

So please indulge me in this fantasy of how that first session might have concluded (a fairly representative example of how Open Dialogue works):

> Because I want to believe in this process, and because I love my family and friends and want to help them, I agree to take a couple of pills, if I don't have to go to hospital.
>
> The doctor says she is comfortable with that, as long as I do take them, and stay away from alcohol, drugs

and stress. She thinks my family need a break from me, and I from them, probably, and she would want to meet again and review how things are going the day after tomorrow.

My partner says she is fine with that, but she worries I won't take the pills, and will lie about it, and get back on the weed and booze as soon as I get home.

Doug suggests he come home with me to make sure I'm OK, and to make sure that there is no weed or alcohol in my flat. I agree to take tonight's pill (quetiapine) in front of him, so he can reassure the others, and another pill tomorrow.

The doctor says she is fine with that, and confirms that we are going to make it two pills across two nights – everyone comfortable with that?

I say I don't see why not – the peer supporter has explained how it helped him, when he was in my shoes.

Yasmin says it would be good if we could all meet again the day after tomorrow, to see how we all are.

My mother is hugely relieved.

My peer supporter is happy that I am calm – my defences have come down a bit, since I don't have to try to argue my way out of being sectioned – and that I am working with the group. He has done good work, as has Yasmin's assistant, as has Yasmin.

Ellie is also relieved that the session has gone so well, and just so happy to see my partner reassured, with the weight of worry and responsibility and isolation visibly lifting off her.

Doug is delighted and he is the sort of person, like everyone here, who likes to help, and he is resolved to assist me and us all through this in any way he can.

Everyone agrees it has been a success. We part with a lot of hugs and tears. We are going to be alright, we say. Maybe not immediately (there's still a lot to deal with and to process) and more meetings and treatments to come, but we all have *hope*.

I really hope you found this section useful, or at least hopeful. Whatever level of care – or deficit of care – you can currently access, it is heartening and comforting that our grandchildren are likely to be treated differently, in line with treatment models with much higher success rates than those we currently endure. But of course I realise that as you read this you are likely to be handling your condition, or that of a sufferer whom you are trying to look after, with nothing like this level of professional support (as we did, and still do).

Although it might not seem as scientific or as medical as a prescription, and though there is nothing like a real Open Dialogue session run by qualified experts, *there is nothing to stop you gathering your network together and trying this sort of approach yourself.* It's only talking and sharing. Being honest and brave in speaking the truth about your fears is surely the hardest thing, but every word and every sentence you can utter, and that someone can hear, is a therapy. We know this because we know that isolation, not talking to anyone, and trying to fight misery and madness yourself, are known to be dangerous and often ineffective: conditions worsen and people die this way.

Everything you are able to share is a lancing of the problem. It may not feel like it at the time – it often doesn't to me – but every truthful sentence expressing your feelings and your needs is a balm, is a salve. You surely have friends like this – people who do not leave the answer to 'How are you?' at 'Fine!' but who are able to say more, maybe much more. The idea that we have to appear 'fine' is a defensive reflex. No one is free from uncertainty.

And so I muddle my way through winter telling my friends I feel rotten and sad and hopeless, and praying that I will come through, and although at the time it often feels as though I am bedding in my depressions by talking about them, talking about them is deeply, palpably helpful to me.

However well you get to know your troubles, you are unlikely to feel great security or certainty about what to expect of them: for good and for ill, health conditions change, life changes, and both change us. One of the lessons I take from Open Dialogue is the idea that in the end we have to make uncertainty a friend. I wish I had known, when I was in my twenties and thirties and early forties, that my uncertainties and fears about jobs I would or would not get, love I might or might not find and money and achievements that I would or would not accrue were as nothing, *nothing*, compared to the certainties I already held. Friendship, meaningful contact, honest love, simple kindness and truth (a big one for someone with as many flaws and self-doubts as me) are the point of it all. Nothing else is certain.

It is surely the case that openness inspires honesty. Admitting vulnerability shows strength, invites confidences and creates solidarity. These are mighty, mighty tools, and they come easier and work ever better with practice. When I teach autobiographical and personal writing, I explain that our first instinct, when exposing ourselves on the page, is to try to put on the best show, to stand in the best light, to conceal those parts of ourselves, our thoughts and deeds about which we have doubts, fears and regrets. But here is the amazing thing. The more open you are, the less you hide, the more you can say, the braver you can be about who you really are, the more, the faster and the more compassionately readers respond to you. It is a leap of faith, not just in ourselves and in our readers, but in humanity. So, how are you, really?

The most important thing about sharing, from a sharing sufferer's point of view (at least in my experience) is the feeling, which grows the more you do it, that you are not the cause of everyone else's worry and fear, and therefore (you feel) responsible for it. You have not chosen to be in trouble. You are an *equal* part of a group, a family, a network of friends, in which you all have problems, you all have stresses and fears and guilts (being human), you all have triggers and raw spots and vulnerabilities.

Remember: *Whatever has happened inside your head is a normal human reaction to whatever has happened to you, and it happens to all of us in some way at some point.*

To trust – and to be given the trust and responsibility and challenge of being part of a network that is trying to make things better for everyone and for you – well, that is no small thing. It's a first step, possibly a big first step, in a good and healthy direction.

8. Going to the doctor

In the first chapters of this book we have looked at ways of thinking, talking about and addressing our problems which have been shown to work. In this section we are going to look at the practicalities: what do you need to know to get the best support, care and self-care? For most of us, distress or mental illness lead us first to a doctor, a general practitioner (GP). I mined my contacts and friends to find one whom I trusted to be absolutely frank about how doctors see us, the sufferers, and our families. When we were at school together, aged seventeen, Kate Chester was a wonderfully sunny, warm person; bright-smiling, she seemed carefree. Now, thirty years later, Dr Kate Kerr retains all her light, her humour and kindness. She looks unchanged. She works – has always worked – extraordinarily hard. Formerly a GP, then a specialist in sexual and reproductive health, Kate now works in the specialist Menopause Clinic at Bath Hospital and at the Royal United Hospital in Bath, seeing both NHS and private patients. When I approached her about contributing to this book she said yes immediately, commenting, 'I see at least one suicidal patient a week.' She asked for some time – she was dealing with another hectic period at work – but soon got back to me, on the last day of her summer holiday, from a rented house in Cornwall. Her husband is also a doctor, working in elderly care, and the couple have two teenaged children.

We connect on the screen and there she is, seaside sunny, wearing a grey top with the word LOVE across it, tanned, relaxed and wonderfully, generously voluble. On the surface she is no one's idea of a ferociously busy clinician, wife and mother. She asks after my mental health: she has kept an eye on me over the years; memorably, she messaged me with concern when my social media posts suggested to her that I might be approaching a manic high. She is reassured, reassuring, and generous with her encouragement of this book. For a moment I see the doctor her patients must see: attentive, listening, looking, her gaze deeply empathetic. Now I explain I want to know what goes through the mind of a doctor, a GP or specialist, when someone first presents themselves in her surgery with a mental health issue.

'The first thing is to make sure they feel validated. It takes a lot of courage to get to this point, to talk to a doctor. They can feel very vulnerable. If they feel fobbed off, at all, it can be exceptionally damaging. After that, in the first minute when they're confessing what they are going through, I don't say anything. As you know, I am a talker! So the first thing I do is listen. It's amazing what comes out in the first minutes. It empowers people to have the chance to say up front what they have to say. And those first minutes can set the whole direction of the consultation.

'And then I prompt them with questions and reflect back what they have said so they know I'm listening.

'And what I'm thinking is, is this person struggling very much? In the current climate everyone is, I don't think anyone's not, but for some it's worse. Everyone has bad runs, mentally, but is this a bad day? A bad week? Has it been going on for a long time?

'A huge percentage of people have fleeting suicidal thoughts – but is this person having them more than usual? So you're thinking, how serious is this? Are they going to hurt themselves or someone else?

'And it sounds awful but as a doctor you're thinking, fucking hell, I'd better not get this wrong. It's quite scary – you might be the last person they say this to, and there will be a massive inquiry if you get it wrong.

'If you think there is a risk they might hurt themselves, you want to find out how active they've been in thinking about suicide. How much structure have they put into their plan? Have they already stockpiled the drugs? Have they started thinking about where they will go to do it? Not that many people have a proper plan, and if they have, then I am worried: I'm thinking, do we need to get hold of a family member? Do we need to get them to a place of safety? Do I need to call the Crisis Team? The on-call psychiatrist? The on-call Community Mental Health Team? (And to be honest you're thinking, fucking hell, this is going to take a lot of time, you're not going to make it to pick your child up from school.) Do they need to be sectioned?'

'And you said you see about one person every week who is thinking of hurting themselves or someone else?' I ask Kate.

'If I had a pound for every menopausal woman who wants to bury her husband under the patio, I'd be rich, but I don't think many of them have done it,' she returns. 'I checked with my GP colleagues, and different areas [of the country] have different templates, but health authorities and Community Mental Health Teams have a protocol-driven system. We use a template. It's good – you're checking a list of symptoms – but then you might lose the connection with someone because you're look-ing at a computer screen. And it really helps us to have a list to hand of all the urgent contacts you might need: the Crisis Team, the on-call psychiatrist, the police – if someone's in danger you might need them to break into someone's home – and the social worker.'

Kate now brings up *an NHS service every reader of this book and everyone concerned with mental health in the UK should know about.* Formerly known as Improving Access to Psychological Therapies (IAPT), the service is now known as NHS Talking Therapies. You will come across IAPT links and references left over from the previous branding. Many links and pages branded IAPT still work. At the time of writing, the national homepage is here:

https://www.nhs.uk/service-search/mental-health/
find-an-nhs-talking-therapies-service

(If the weblink changes, you'll be able to find NHS Talking Therapies via a web search.)

This is the national, overall page. If you or someone close to you is in trouble, you will need the one in your area. The page has a 'Start now' button. Click it and you are told that you are self-referring (this is a good thing: you're putting the system to work) and that the service will contact you, and that you will be recommended a therapy. Click the 'Continue' button and you are asked for the name or road name of your GP surgery. Put it in, select your surgery, and things start to happen: an IAPT page comes up, with a link to self-refer. A phone number for IAPT services comes up: call it and you are through to NHS Talking Therapies for Anxiety and Depression. Contact numbers and emails for your local mental health hospital also come up (for example, the hospital where I was treated) along with a reassurance that you can self-refer. There is also a 'refer yourself online' button which puts you through to Vita Health Group, a private provider contracted by the NHS. It offers a fairly cheap-looking website which, nevertheless, provides an accurate and useful list of services, from OCD Action to Bereavement Care, Depression Alliance, Mind and No More Panic. (It may seem fairly typical of Britain that a private company is being paid to make the link between your overworked GP and these excellent, life-saving charities, but there we are.)

The important point is that you can self-refer and it is

not difficult to do. (You can do it for a friend or loved one, with their permission.) And the thing to know is, these are the same numbers and the same services your GP uses, whether you are an NHS or private patient. NHS Talking Therapies / IAPT is a crucial, invaluable place to start, and a key part of your treatment, recovery and healing journey.

Kate uses it all the time. As she says, 'People can find out for themselves the local contacts you need in a crisis. You can find out how to self-refer. As you know, people are now waiting up to three weeks for a GP appointment. They might ring the surgery and get through to reception, who tell them to call back in the morning at eight, and then we've missed the window and someone harms themselves, and it's absolutely awful. The thing that goes through my head is, I need to help you take responsibility a bit. It really is Step One of your healing. In the darkest period you may not be able to do anything, but when you can, it really empowers you to begin to take charge of your condition.'

In order to explore this more fully, and thinking of my students at the University of Manchester, and of myself when I was their age, I present Kate with a hypothetical case study.

'Supposing I ring the doctor and get an appointment with you. I'm severely depressed. I haven't made practical plans to end my life but I'm so miserable I just wish I didn't exist. What do you do? What will happen to me? What will you say to me?'

Kate does not hesitate. You can tell, listening to her and watching her on the screen, that this is reflex, core territory for her. As she says later, which brings me up short so that I get her to repeat it, *over half of the people doctors see are presenting with a mental health issue.*

'Validation first. I tell you that asking for help is a brave thing and you are doing the right thing – just being here, you have done the right thing. If you're a young person, I'll tell you how common this is. That you are at the most common age for this to happen to you.

'Then we'll talk about the talking therapies. We'll work out whether you are going to go NHS or self-funded.'

I had the same experience – the doctor, crisis team member or psychiatrist gives you an idea of how long the waiting list for therapy is, what you can access when your turn finally comes, and enquires, delicately, whether you can afford to go private. Appointments with therapists cost anything from £60 an hour upwards: there are plenty of people out there paying more than double this, too.

Kate continues, 'We talk through different options in therapies. We will discuss whether this is an acute anxiety that seems temporary, or is it a bit more long term? And, depending, we will talk about medication. If you need medication, I explain how the different drugs work. I will be aiming to take away any fear you might have. I will explain the side effects of different medications. I will talk about dosages and how long they take to work. And I'll ask, what are you going to do with yourself if it takes three weeks for the medication to start taking effect? What support networks do you have? What is your lifestyle, and how can you change it to improve your situation?

'And if you're a twenty-one year old – especially if you're a 21-year-old bloke! – what are you taking? Are you drinking? Are you taking drugs? Do you exercise? What about your contacts with other human beings?

'Because you know the reality is that NHS services are not going to cut it, often, because of the waiting times.'

Waiting times vary from one NHS trust to another, and from one therapy to another. To take a random and illustrative example, if you receive a referral for cognitive behavioural therapy (CBT) in Leeds you will be told the waiting time is currently 14 months. National NHS targets require that 75 per cent of patients should be able to access therapy within 6 weeks of referral, and 95 per cent within 18 weeks. But NHS data collected and analysed by the leading mental health charity Mind suggests that 1 in 10 people have been waiting over a year to receive treatment; over half have been waiting over 3 months, and around 13 per cent of people are still waiting for their first assessment for psychological therapy. You can see why people who can afford it tend to go private. There are also plenty of us who cannot really afford it, but who make cuts, savings and sacrifices in order to buy therapy for ourselves or those we love.

When a GP like Kate has a patient who cannot afford to go private, their next move is to look at what is available on NHS Talking Therapies / IAPT, and how long are the waiting lists. Next, they look at which charities and organisations in the local area might be able to help.

'I'm making an assessment about when this needs to be followed up. It's likely to be two weeks, but it's all about individualisation, isn't it? Is this a new condition? Or is it chronic? Each person's experience and the support they need is different. I'm trying to work out what makes you tick. And a lot of our role, as health professionals, is signposting.'

Aware that Kate works too hard, and this is the last day of her summer holiday, I limit myself to two more questions.

'It sounds as though you have all the tools you need to treat mental health. So can someone who is in mental distress be confident that the doctor can really help them? Have you *got* this? Can the system we have contain the trouble people might get into, and help them heal?'

Kate hesitates. 'In theory, yes. A lot of things are very treatable. That's why it's such a failure of the system when someone does take their own life. Most GPs are people who really care. My private work allows me to be the doctor I want to be, to really take the time, so they can pour their heart out and I have the time to bring them back. But on the NHS in ten minutes? You do your best. You're a hope-giver, that's the thing. And in a GP practice you might have one doctor who is a heart specialist, and one who is really good at giving knee injections, and someone who is the Mental Health Lead, or Men's Health, or Women's Health Lead. With mental health we aim to listen, validate, communicate, empower and signpost. It's unusual to just prescribe: the question is, what are you going to do to adapt your life?

'But doctors are human beings too. You might get a GP on a bad day. They might have something happening at home. Or you might find you didn't quite gel. So you can ask, do you have someone here who is the Mental Health Lead? No one is going to mind you asking that question. Or you can shop around – you can go outside the practice, and ask around: who's good, who's not?'

During the period after my breakdown, when I was shaky and uncertain, and frightened of medication, I rather avoided my local surgery. It never occurred to me that there are other practices in the Calder Valley, that I could have 'shopped around', as Kate put it, and sought out specialist mental health GPs, or those who are particularly adept with mental health problems. I had no idea that this was even possible. But Kate is adamant: if she or someone close to her was in trouble, this is exactly what she would do.

'We're seeing a lot of people in the darkest places, and we see them managing their ups and downs and other ups – *everyone* is living on the spectrum of mental health, they're lying if they say they're not. But you will learn more about yourself, whatever age you are, you're not a robot, you're an evolving being. If it's not working, start thinking about making some changes, realistic changes. It really is about self-empowerment.

'And there is a lot to be hopeful about, there really is. People come to me now and talk about their diagnoses, and their treatment plans. I tell them never to make instant decisions. Always sleep on it. Read up on it. Read books! Do the best you can.'

Finally, I ask Dr Kate Kerr about her own work, and how she manages her own mental health.

'I have really chosen carefully and cherry-picked what I wanted to do with my career. (I don't know how long I will keep it up: I might retire and open a coffee van! But hopefully my husband won't ...) Working as a menopause specialist, I see a lot of mental health – forty-five to fifty-five is the age when women are most likely to take their own lives. I use the Balance app in my work a lot, it's excellent (www.balance-menopause.com/balance-app/). If you're interested, you should look at the work of Dr Louise Newson, she is super-bright, just brilliant; you can find her work on YouTube and the web. You can really help someone with the menopause, with Hormone Replacement Therapy but also other ways. Not necessarily Husband Replacement Therapy!

'For me I take regular breaks. I am selective about what I do with my time off. I go on holiday without mates, just with a book. I walk a lot, I run twice a week. My husband and I both noticed we were drinking more, so now I do three nights a week with no alcohol. Once a week I play tennis. The coffee after is the most important mental health time of my week – I have a really close group of girlfriends and our chats then, that's when it all gets sorted out. There will often be one of us who needs something and there are always ways we can help each other. And I love London. Because I trained there it's such a happy place for me. Sometimes I just go to London and sit in a café . . .'

We say our goodbyes. I sit back and take a moment. Kate is a palpably caring and competent person. Were I or anyone I loved in trouble, I would seek her out. Our system is full of people like her, who work furiously hard, against vicious pressures, and who care deeply, and who wish they had more time and more resources in order to give more care. I found talking to her hugely helpful and reassuring, and something more than that – I found what she told me inspiring. The system *does* have a vast reservoir of good and effective treatments and contacts to offer.

Rule 9: Accessing what you need when you need it will be work, perhaps hard and frustrating work. But know the help is out there.

9. Common maladies:
Dope and hope

The most upsetting thing I have heard while researching this subject was something an Approved Mental Health Professional (a specialist social worker) said when I interviewed her about sectioning me, and about her profession. Months after I had come out of the psychiatric hospital, during the period of recovery, we met on an afternoon of sun and rain in an office in Halifax, and spoke for a long time about her work. We covered my case, and the way she thinks about helping people in trouble, and how and why detaining people is done. (Social workers hate the term 'sectioning', she said; they prefer 'detain'.) And then we talked more generally about how professionals like her view the currents of mental health.

She said, 'Christmas is a nightmare, obviously, with a great rise in crises and distress, and big football matches and tournaments.' (Nurses, doctors and police officers all say the same thing: football, alcohol, domestic violence and mental trauma are old friends.) And then she said the thing that scared me, 'And of course the under thirties suffer from everything.'

And she meant it. She did not mean the young are flaky or weak. She meant that they are assailed by pressures on their well-being, by traumas and distresses, and that you can find every condition which hurts and damages people causing hurt and damage to the young.

Visit any town, any university, and you will see that in terms of material things – tech, clothes, phones, apps – the young of the West are among the most privileged generations who have ever lived. They are also among the most vulnerable in our society to personal, economic and social shocks; they are on the wrong side of our divided society (though many have wealthy parents and networks, many more do not); and perhaps above all, at this age and stage of life, people are deeply sensitive to the currents and pressures of the time.

A landmark study funded by the Economic and Social Research Council and undertaken by the Sutton Trust and University College London found that:

> . . . almost half (44%) of young people were above the threshold for 'probable mental ill health', using the General Health Questionnaire (GHQ-12), indicating high levels of psychological distress. This has increased dramatically from 35% in 2017 and 23% in 2007 (from previous cohort studies looking at similar ages), point- ing to a decline in the mental health and wellbeing of young people, likely accelerated by the pandemic.

Furthermore, the study found:

Those who identify as female report elevated psycho- logical distress (54%), self-harm (23%) and suicide attempts (11%), compared to those who identify as male (33% report distress, 11% report self-harm and 5% report attempting suicide). Overall, 8% of participants reported that they had ever attempted to end their life. This figure is comparable with data from 2017 (7%).

This study is the largest of its kind into the impact of the pandemic on young people. It may be that the questionnaire focused respondents' minds on how the pandemic made them feel, and anyone who knows a young person will know it was an especially brutal time for them, mentally, which came at an especially vulnerable stage of life. As we will see when we look at anxiety, modern life is particularly adept at producing future threats that we can be sure we will face, from escalating costs and increasing competition for resources to climate change and pandemics associated with increased and ageing populations. It is not so good at producing reassurances that we as individuals and families will be able to cope. As in first love or first heartbreak, early experiences of mental distress are particularly awful. You have nothing with which to compare what you are experiencing. You may have no idea why it is happening to you, and you have no idea if it will end. It can feel as though your life to come will be a trial of madness and misery.

Leaving aside the indictment of our society that the suffering of the young represents, what kind of world have we built, that they should 'suffer from everything'? Let us look at what can help.

Normalisation

The first point is normalisation, which is particularly pointed and important in the case of a student, for example. I worked with Mark Oakley, the Dean of Chapel at St John's College, Cambridge, on a series of fifteen-minute films called *What Really Matters,* which he intended to be of use and help to Cambridge students, especially undergraduates, and especially with their mental health. The thoughtful and sensitive young people who become Cambridge students suffer – as a great many thoughtful and sensitive young people do, at university or outside it – from a range of mental health conditions, from anxiety and insomnia through to eating disorders, depression and breakdown. So although a first encounter with mental suffering may well make you feel as though you have been singled out, and that there is something fundamentally wrong with you, the truth is that experiencing mental ill health at a young age puts you in a very sizeable section of the population. You are unlucky but you are not in any way abnormal. Rates change constantly, but NHS data drawn from a three-wave study which began in 2017 and ran until 2022 shows that 18 per cent of children aged seven to sixteen years and 22 per cent of young people aged seventeen to twenty-four years had a probable mental disorder.

So as a young person, you should *expect* to encounter mental health troubles, either in yourself or in the people around you. Statistically, you will. The student body as a whole has a high rate of mental health difficulties. Whatever your subject, whether you are in university or college or not, if you are young, you are vulnerable. In fact, your vulnerability speaks volumes for you: it is a function of being a sensitive, creative and caring person, with hopes, desires, fears and dreams.

It is worth remembering that we make demands of the young that adults almost never make of each other. I can't remember hearing one of my older friends ask another, 'So what do you plan to do with your life? What job/plan/subject are you going to pursue? What would you like to be doing in five years' time?' Most of us have only the vaguest idea of how to respond to these questions, yet our culture makes the young feel inadequate if they cannot answer them.

Making sense of it: Why are you in trouble?

The first time I hit depression, in the second year of university, I did not know what it was. I thought I was going mad with unhappiness. I was fairly sure it was all my fault, too:

I had fallen out with a lot of my friends, over a relationship.
I had not done much work, and was behind.

My reaction to freedom, to responsibility for myself and my own time, had been to smoke as much dope as possible.

Dope made me happy and lazy: I got further behind and became more isolated. (My idea of a Saturday night was to get extremely stoned and go to the chip van.)

I did not know what an English degree was even for: what was the point of it?

I felt guilty for the time and money (state money, in those days, and mine, and my father's) which I had wasted, smoked and spent.

I had profound doubts about my own worth and place in the world: what was I for? What was I going to do?

I was completely blank and rather terrified at the thought of life after university: how did anyone ever afford a car, never mind a house?

Jobs, as one of my few remaining friends, a fellow English student, put it, seemed to be a choice between jobs you couldn't ever get and jobs you would rather die than do. Even aside from the misery I felt, the future looked shit.

I didn't feel much respect for the university, for other students, for (John Major's) Britain (which had many of exactly the same problems and unnecessary cruelties as this one), for capitalism, for the West, for human beings, or for myself. It seemed to me that the rich were going to get richer, the poor get poorer, that inequality was here to stay, that the fortunate enjoyed a great wealth of opportunity, and that the unfortunate were condemned to struggle, and that no politician was going to have much success with making real change, even supposing they wanted to.

My workload was absolutely on top of me: there was no way I could both meet all my deadlines and turn in good or even decent essays.

I had been trying out Class A drugs, including amphetamines, cocaine, MDMA and ecstasy, which had wiped out my bank balance and further alienated me from my friends (when I get high I go very high, and act like a dick, or a nutter, or both).

I was in debt, both to the Student Loans Company and the bank.

My flatmates thought I was a complete twat, because I was. (It was mutual, but they were right.)

I was looking at leaving with a very poor or indifferent degree, in serious debt, and heading into a world I was unprepared for: who wants to hire some git with a lame English degree, a serious cannabis habit, no money, no mates, no contacts, no practical knowledge and no skills?

I was a broke, odd, miserable, lonely, druggy weirdo, in my own frank estimation.

I did not know it, but I was carrying a great weight laid down in my childhood, a weight of insecurity, perfectionism, and deep doubts about my own self-worth. If you are suffering from mental ill health, the chances are the roots of it are in your childhood, too, as any decent therapist will tell you.

Many, many students I have taught and worked with in the last ten years have been in some or all of these situations, though they have always seemed much braver and more graceful about it than I was.

It is no wonder at all that young people get depressed, or anxious, or suffer from insomnia, or eating disorders, or self-harm, or a combination of these. It makes absolute sense: these are understandable, normal and entirely reasonable responses to the state of education, to the state of higher education in many places, to the state of the nation and the world.

The psychological pressures exerted on the young by capitalism, social media, the media, the economy, the climate crisis, and by local, national and global inequality, and our culture – which still places the old and comfortable in charge, and gives them the power to organise the world to best suit them, at the expense of the young – are, objectively, brutal.

We should *expect* many people in this situation to react as they do: by retreating into online life, by reaching for drugs and alcohol.

Normal response: Cannabis

Although there is noise in the media about Gen Z being less drawn to drink and drugs than previous generations, the statistics show that:

- 38 per cent of fifteen year olds have taken drugs
- 19 per cent of sixteen to twenty-four year olds have used cannabis in the last year
- 89 per cent of young people who seek medical help with issues related to drugs are cannabis users.

If you are very lucky, strong and sensible, you may have avoided cannabis altogether, and I salute your strength and your choices. But I feel it is worth knowing about the damage it can do and understanding ways of dealing with it – you surely have or will meet friends along the way who have got into it, and rare indeed is the parent or grandparent whose children, grandchildren and their friends have avoided it.

Why do we – dope smokers – do it? (Although I now avoid cannabis, it took being sectioned to teach me to stop, and part of me will always be a dope addict.)

At first it is wonderful. Colours are brighter, sounds are richer, thoughts are more intriguing, exciting and moving. In my case, everything I see and hear and think seems shot through with deeper meanings than when I am straight. Everything has more resonance: suddenly you are not a stoned student meandering about the suburbs of York on a dreary winter night in 1994; you are a poet walking through East Berlin in the 1960s one second, and a traveller in the whole glittering wide universe the next. It makes me funnier and more insightful (or so I feel), and my friends, too. We spent about three university terms, the whole of first year, making each other giggle like kids. I did not think I would ever have more joyous times than the best I have had while stoned on cannabis – and, given the way it raises levels of serotonin and dopamine in the brain, this was technically true for a long time. And so it is not surprising that people who smoke a lot of dope soon move from getting high with friends to getting high alone.

I dedicated so much time to it, so much money and so much energy. I could have learned two or three languages in the time I put into dope. I could have saved up enough money to travel the world, start a pension, accumulate the deposit for a house or buy a car. Had it not been for the disastrous and torturous consequences for my mental health, and the chaotic destruction I wrought on my life, relationships and career, and the cruel, scourging costs to people who loved me, and whom I love, I would not have regretted it at all. Alcohol was never my thing. Dope was my thing.

Savage failings in policy and public information are responsible for the ambiguity that still surrounds cannabis. It is worth making the point unambiguously: cannabis is responsible for appalling levels of mental suffering, from anxiety and paranoia (which many long-term smokers are guaranteed) to depression (few of my friends who smoked heavily escaped this) and psychosis.

And there is a divide between generations' experience of weed: while in the nineties we had fairly light hash, mostly, my students have much stronger varieties. While the levels of THC I was getting were around 2–5 per cent, THC levels are massively higher now: 20–25 per cent.

In terms of the smoking experience, a light sweet block of old-fashioned Moroccan, what I think of as 'high happy hash', is a world away from a joint packed with skunk. It's the difference between light ale and home-brewed, moonshine vodka. Smoking dope, now, is much more like taking acid than getting stoned. As a result, psychosis and schizophrenia among cannabis users are much more common this century than last. One of our most eminent and experienced psychiatrists, Sir Robin Murray, reports that a third of his patients with psychosis are suffering because of cannabis.

Robin is married to Marta Di Forti, an expert on the drug's effects, who runs a cannabis psychosis support group based in the Maudsley Hospital, London. There is huge demand for her service, but no funding. While government policy and the national conversation admit only a hazy, anecdotal link between cannabis, depression and psychosis, no expert, no sufferer and no sufferer's family is in any doubt whatsoever.

Dealing with the consequences of cannabis

While cannabis floods the brain with dopamine and serotonin, it also damages the systems which produce these neurotransmitters. I found I needed more joints to get the same euphoric feelings, and then, when I stopped (late in second year, the first time – it felt like the moment to try to rescue my degree), down I went.

Feelings of hopelessness, panic, an inability to concentrate, social paranoia and anxiety, crushing shame and stinging guilt, insomnia, an inability to remember anything, and overwhelming feelings of fear led me to feel I just did not want to exist any more. I did not deserve to exist, I felt. I thought about suicide a lot. I did not plan it in any meaningful way, but I longed not to be alive.

As far as I could tell, and according to the evidence which was my life and my feelings at that time, I had smoked myself into a state of misery and stupidity, destroying my brain and my life chances.

I went to a doctor and begged him to do something. I would have taken anything to make my misery and panic go away. Prozac was popular at the time, and I asked for a prescription.

He said, 'So, you've been addicted to cannabis, you've quit, you're miserable, and now you want Prozac? I don't think so.'

I could have hit him – he had a blond bristly face and I remember wanting to punch it – but I owe him a tremendous amount. Instead of intervening, bluntly and chemically, in my battered brain, he sent me away to deal with the consequences myself.

Today, doctors and psychiatrists are far more ready to

prescribe antidepressants to young people, and to everyone, than was that doctor. I wish I could thank him personally.

I am not, incidentally, anti-cannabis. I see it as a balance between health and choice. A massive public information campaign about its dangers; decriminalisation; selling it in shops, accurately and truthfully labelled with THC levels, and expert tasting notes, as it were, detailing each strain's effects; all these might help. We do it with wine, after all. I would like to see people having a wide and clear choice between different strengths and strains, and I would prohibit it to the under twenty-ones on the grounds of brain development. My students at the University of Manchester tell me that they distinguish between different strains and have access to different varieties in a way that my generation did not: everyone should have access to clear and accurate information on what they are choosing to smoke. When it comes to my family and close friends among the young, my advice is: hold off as much as possible, be as old as possible, smoke the lightest possible. If it were up to me, we would legalise it, and every pack would say: Cannabis is commonly associated with anxiety, depression, psychosis and schizophrenia. *Use very sparingly*.

So, when you stop cannabis, although some people come off it with no problems, others can expect variations of all the miseries outlined above, and your own particular torments. What should you do?

Know that your misery and panic do end. Your

serotonin and dopamine systems have taken a battering but they are still there. You WILL feel better. You WILL feel as happy, in the future, off dope, as you did before you used it. You WILL laugh as loudly and feel as blissful, in the future, without weed, as you did during your best highs.

Know that your intelligence and ability are still there. I wrote my essays in third year, one appalled, hopeless word at a time, not knowing how my sentences would end, unable to come up with or remember good ideas, unable to take in what I read. It was a shitshow, honestly. But fifteen books later, not all of them that bad, my writing career is proof that the brain can and does come through. (I moved on to skunk and smoked on and off for decades, including hundreds of pipes, bongs and buckets, so don't go thinking that if you are young and have been into high-strength weed you must have done more smoking-brain-damage than me. You definitely haven't.)

Know that time is on your side. The unbeatable ally, the power behind you which no power can match, is time. Every day you stay off, you increase the chances and speed the process of recovery. According to neuroscience, your brain is still developing. As Sarah-Jayne Blakemore, Professor of Psychology and Cognitive Neuroscience at the University of Cambridge, has put it:

> The brain continues to develop through childhood and adolescence and even into the 20s and 30s in some brain regions. White matter increases, grey matter

decreases. These changes are thought to be caused by important neurodevelopmental processes that enable the brain to be moulded and influenced by the environment.

So you see, it is ALL still to play for.

Dr Marta Di Forti of King's College London, mentioned above, runs an intervention scheme. She told cannabishealthnews.co.uk:

We have under our care at any given time, between 240 and 300 patients at the beginning of psychosis and 45–50 per cent have come to the first stage of psychosis from cannabis. I'm not saying that for all of them cannabis is the main factor, because they come from a history of trauma, as well as poverty, migration and other complications – there are a pool of risk factors. But certainly when they are able to reduce [their cannabis use] or they change the way they use it, or for those who want to, stop completely, you do see a significant improvement.

Accept that the way out is less fun (possibly a hell of a lot less) than the way in, but there *is* a way, and you can take it. For me, the first couple of weeks after stopping were miserable. The second couple were better. Weeks five and six I really started to come round. This has been the pattern with me ever since that first inundating depression. You will have your own pattern, but there is a lot you can do to aid time's healing.

You are giving your system a chance to rebalance. You can help it with diet and exercise, of course. New activities do work. 'If we could give them in pill form, nature and exercise,' said one consultant psychiatrist I interviewed, 'would be among the most powerful drugs we have.' But this is all very well in theory. I tended to feel too depressed to face anything, never mind bloody exercise. Nevertheless, the facts are clear – exercise is good for our bodies and minds. If you can find somewhere pleasant to walk, cycle, run or swim, it's good for the soul, too.

Change your circumstances. If your feelings are your outputs, then your situation, your days, whatever you put into your body, and the place in which you find yourself, are your inputs. So *change them*.

We descend from nomads. Research cited by BBC Radio 4's excellent *All in the Mind* suggests that we need changing horizons to be happy. So even if the idea of a run appals you (it surely does me), take a walk to a new part of town or wherever you are. If you find yourself on a miserable ring road, a bleak suburb or an ugly agri-industrial wasteland, and go home wet and tired and feeling worse, at least you have had some exercise. You have taken action. You have taken control and made a move. You are beginning to be the master of your fate. *(I do not know of any way through any mental health condition that does not involve taking control of your own healing.)*

If you cannot give up right away, take control of your habit. In Morocco, where cannabis has been smoked for centuries, dope smokers have evolved a socially acceptable and relatively safe system for most people, depending on genetic vulnerability. If you really must, have a light one after your evening meal and perhaps, if you really want to, have one more before you go to bed: this is how the people of the High Atlas do it, one of them told me – and they've been smoking it for centuries.

I would steer the hell away from the strong stuff. As you cut your usage your tolerance goes down and you get the same kick, anyway. Plus, light usage boosts dopamine, while heavy smoking depresses it. So if you want to feel better and have more fun, smoke lightly.

The Canigma website offers this excellent list of recommendations in an article by Janelle Lassalle, for mitigating side effects:

- Avoid mixing dope with stimulants (alcohol, caffeine, nicotine) as these can exacerbate the negative effects of cannabis. For example, small amounts of alcohol can significantly increase the amount of THC – the psychoactive ingredients responsible for the cannabis high – in the blood.
- Exercise! Walking, yoga, dance, sport and swimming are all good for your health, your well-being and your state of mind. I am a great fan of cold water swimming, and when that goes beyond cold to hell-freezing, in the Yorkshire winter, I take a cold shower daily, until the ice melts.

- Deep breathing exercises ('diaphragmatic breathing') can help ease the discomfort of racing or anxious thoughts.
- Listening to uplifting or calming music.

Addiction and despair

While I began writing this book with a great sense of purpose and optimism, and in a generally very happy and fortunate-feeling place, that blessed state only lasted so long. Although the fundamentals were strong, and remain so – my dear ex and I are on excellent terms; our boy is happy and well – the end of the year, the failure of a relationship which seemed to promise the world but did not work out (mostly due to my myriad inadequacies and complexes), the coming of the winter, worries about everything (health and happiness of loved ones, work, bills, the future, the state of the world, you name it) took me into a hard place.

It does not matter how many times you go there and come out of it, or how firmly you tell yourself (for you know it, you've proved it) that it *does* end, despair feels like the final, desperate end of all hope. Lathered in self-loathing and chin-deep in fear, you have to fight yourself to do everything, from getting up in the morning onwards.

Around this time I took the advice of a wise friend, who said that it was ludicrous that I should attempt to write a useful book about mental health without trying one of the most powerful and widespread options available to anyone who is suffering, and who has ever been addicted to anything – AA (Alcoholics Anonymous) or NA (Narcotics Anonymous).

Although I have definitely drunk too much over the course of my life so far – and, in bursts, spectacularly too much – I don't identify as someone who has a problem with alcohol. I can stop for months on end without difficulty or craving. (Advancing age seems to make me more sleepy than thirsty now, after a couple, which I definitely did not see coming. The amount of trouble my previously fearsome second wind has got me into over the years does not bear thinking about.) And I have definitely been addicted to cannabis, but not used it more than once or twice in the past five years, and not missed it. Therefore, I told my friend, I did not think AA or NA were for me.

I was also a bit suspicious, because one of my friends was a dedicated AA attendee and it seemed to take up a lot of her life, and I was not convinced that returning to drinking would have been especially dangerous for her: the behaviours she described, when she was drinking, were a long way from the downward spiral of the chronic alcoholic. But part of the Twelve Steps programme upon which AA is built is the spreading of the good news of sobriety and freedom from addiction, through AA, to others.

I wondered whether my friend was fulfilling a

missionary duty in recruiting me, as it were, for her own reasons as much as for mine?

Now I am sure she was not. As she explained, once an addict, always an addict. Had I not transferred my addictive needs to other things than cannabis – relationships, sex, cigarettes?

Indeed I had.

Didn't I think that being a drug addict for so long must have long-term consequences? The lying, the deceit, the damage to self and others?

Indeed I do.

Did I understand that going to an NA meeting did not have to be about having a drug addiction now, but about the consequences of having been addicted for so long?

This one took me longer to accept. I kept saying, 'But I haven't smoked (like that) for years!'

To which she replied, 'So what? I haven't drunk for years. But I still go to a meeting every week!'

In the depths of that miserable winter, I went. Partly to find out, and partly because I was in a bad place, lacking the courage to attend Andy's Man Club (a suicide prevention group for men which has gently spectacular results, and which I unreservedly recommend, having researched the heck out of it, while still lacking the courage to attend) but desperate to talk to and be heard by *somebody*.

(I also spent ages looking up the Samaritans online, and have their number saved in my phone, although I have yet to use it.)

It was a normal vile Yorkshire winter night, rain spattering like black grease, cold and dirty-feeling. I walked to the station and took the train to a nearby town, hoping I would not see anybody I knew. Outside the meeting place a group of a dozen or so people had gathered. They were talking and laughing loudly, waiting to go in. I hid behind a bush and had a cigarette, feeling that I could never be part of such a group (being too shit, personality-wise, and my confidence too low). And then the doors opened, and they went in. I swore at myself and followed.

The rules of AA/NA, which your attendance signals your willingness to follow, include the promise that what you see, hear and say will not leave the room. Thus I am only going to describe what happened in the most general terms, in the hope that something here might be useful. Addiction, after all, is a mighty driver of misery and mental suffering, and whatever else you might think of or hear about AA/NA, they have been dealing with it for a very long time, to the benefit, they would argue, of millions. AA puts its current membership at over two million, with 75 per cent in the US and Canada. It started in 1935, in Ohio, when a stockbroker and a surgeon who had both recovered from alcoholism met and began to hold meetings and draw up the book of case histories and steps to recovery which became the foundation of Alcoholics Anonymous.

It was a small room with a circle of chairs, with a kettle and cups by a sink. As soon as I walked in people turned to me and smiled. No big deal was made. A kindly man said hello, welcome. I did not have many words – I was struggling with all kinds of communication – and so I sat down. The others in the room seemed very happy to see each other, the atmosphere was like a group of colleagues meeting outside work, perhaps for some sort of event or away-day. They were all aware of me (I suspect I lugged a weight of fear-filled, paranoid anti-energy in with me, something which felt to me like the putrefying corpse of a bubonic plague-killed bison) but they were careful not to show it, not to make me feel singled out or different. It was very touching, as though the basic philosophies of this group were sensitivity and a gentle kindness.

I kept looking for the leader, the authority figure, but although one man emerged as the person who would be running the session, in the sense of keeping us to time, and making a couple of announcements, no one was in charge, in the conventional sense.

One of my fears, which seems pathetic now, was that I would be laughed at, secretly or overtly, for being a lightweight, for not having been sufficiently addicted to sufficiently dangerous or powerful drugs. A few years of dope-smoking, a posh voice and a comfy middle-class life; who the hell did I think I was? I knew this town, like many towns in the North-West, had real problems with heroin and other Class A narcotics. I felt ashamed of having got myself into such a mess, for such a long time, from a background of intellectual, professional and educational privilege, with something which I felt was relatively mild.

It was a nonsense fear, of course, and though I held on to it through the session, the atmosphere, right from the outset, made me feel – made me sure – that this was not a place of judgement, much less unkind judgement. The group were men, women and non-binary, and a great range of ages. And they really were happy to be there, to see each other. There was something (I cannot put this any better) lovely about it.

So I sat there feeling like a mute fraud. And then something happened which I will never forget. The man who had first said hello to me came and sat next to me, on my right. And at the same time, as if it were choreographed, another man, of similar age to me and the first man, came and sat on my left. They both said hello, and their names, and we shook hands. And for a moment that was that. But it was extraordinary. Despite daily contact with my family, and all sorts of conversations and meetings with people I was working with, and regular phone calls with friends and my mum, and despite brief contact most days with people in town, from my friends who work in shops to acquaintances who also use them, I had been utterly, desperately lonely for weeks. But I only knew quite how lonely I had been when those two strangers sat down on either side of me. It was in the way they did it, I think: their immediate choice to sit there, to flank and support me, without words, when there were a dozen other seats they could have picked, and places next to other people they clearly knew and liked – it was really something. By that simple action they seemed to be saying, 'We're in this with you.' And the strangest thing was, I could *feel* their support. I could actually physically feel it, as if I had been very cold and someone had placed a radiator on either side of me.

After the greeting they went back to engaging with the room, not looking at me especially, but I sat there as if astonishingly bathed in warmth. I felt like I grew an inch in every direction, and in my soul, in those moments. It was their instinctive decision to take up positions of support, and what they must have been thinking as they did it (something along the lines of, 'This poor sod could do with a bit of help,' I imagine), and the fact, which I had never realised so plainly before, which I had only glimpsed in lovers, or in someone who wanted to fight me, that you can actually feel people's feelings towards you, in the same plain way you feel rain or wind or a draught.

It was like magic. I wish I could give that feeling to everyone who is suffering, and everyone who will suffer. This may seem over the top but I was in a raw, scared place, and that moment was the nearest thing I have experienced to whatever the Bible means by being filled with the Holy Spirit.

The session began. You have probably seen mock-ups in films or on TV of similar sessions. People say their names, followed by, 'I'm an addict,' and are answered by name with a greeting from the group. You don't have to give your real name, of course. They share a story – mostly of how they have been doing, how they are getting on, what's coming up for them, in the case of this group. The convention is, no one refers back to what they have heard or directly responds to it – this is called 'cross-sharing', and it is not done, so you are heard without judgement or comment.

I could not bring myself to 'share', or to say the sacred – to AA and NA – words, 'I am an addict.' The group did not ask me to, explicitly, but they made a space in which I could have done, had I been strong enough. When they realised it was my first ever session they were particularly attentive. They praised my courage (which I did not feel I possessed) in coming to the session, and some commented, in their shares, on their first time – how lost they were before, and how much better they felt, how much stronger and less lost they were now.

The most striking thing about all of them, and they were a great variety of people, was how honest and genuine they seemed. There is something powerfully attractive about an individual who is prepared to admit vulnerability, fallibility and disastrous life choices (if they really were choices, given the trauma it was easy to imagine in some of their backgrounds), and however different we were, and despite whatever we might have felt about one another in other contexts, in this context we liked and trusted each other. We had faith in each other.

And they were very happy to be there, that was the

other obvious thing. Despite the stories of pain and damage from which they had emerged, which they were still coping with, it was a quietly joyous session – there was warmth and laughter; feelings of productivity and progress attended every moment. I imagine this is because each member of the group is, in therapeutic terms, both client and therapist. We were all helping each other and being helped just by being there.

The mantra of the session was 'Just for today' – just for today I am not using. One person had an anniversary, a certain number of days of being off drugs, and we celebrated that. Addicts in recovery, like the elite soldiers of the Parachute Regiment and the Special Air Service, achieve their aims by setting small achievable goals: one minute, one hour, one day at a time. They gave me a key ring with the phrase 'Just for today' on it, and, most movingly, they gave me – these strangers, who knew nothing about me whatsoever – their personal mobile phone numbers, so that should I need to, I could call on any of them for support.

When I went home I knew I would not go again, and I would not call any of those numbers. I felt that if I had been in the grip of addiction at the time it would have been a wonderful, perhaps lifesaving choice, to keep going to the sessions, to follow the steps, to take the support that was offered. But I was not in that place, and I did not feel I could give it all the time it would ask of me.

The experience led me to urge AA on two people,

friends, both of whom struggle with booze. One felt that AA was not for him. Instead he took time off, dried himself out and returned to a relationship with drink which is much better balanced – he still drinks, but he no longer lurches from bender to hangover and back. The other went to AA. He decided not to follow the whole Twelve Steps but he did find it helped, along with other changes he made, to bring him to a much better place: eighteen months after his time of desperate despair I heard from his partner that he was back on a much more even keel.

Both sufferers made the same moves. First they got in touch with someone whom they knew would understand, who had been in a similar place and who would not judge them, known in recovery as a 'peer supporter'. I did not need to have been an alcoholic to be their peer supporter; the facts of my also having broken down, hit the bottom, and come through, were enough. And they both refused to let feelings of misery, regret, hopelessness and despair shame them into silence. They spoke out, asked for help, looked for ways forward, and then took them. A combination of actions like this – simple to outline, simple to do once you start, but hard to start – *does work*. Which leads us to Rule 10:

Rule 10: The Addiction Monster, as some therapists call it, is infinitely beatable. It feeds on silence and shame – so speak out. It feeds on solitude – so find a peer supporter. It feeds on inertia – so act.

To be surrounded by peer supporters, which is the effect of walking into an AA or NA meeting, to be trusted and treated as though you are brave and good and admirable, is truly wonderful, and truly remarkable when you are feeling like a worthless mess. I would recommend absolutely anyone go to AA or NA for that experience. As well as being extraordinarily successful, the networks are free and available everywhere, every week. Alcoholics Anonymous puts its worldwide membership at over two million people; these are long-term recovering drinkers who are fully involved in the programme. At the level of individual visits, people who may go a few times, or just once, like me, the numbers jump – three million people in the UK alone.

The fact that the meetings are free, and that you are unlikely to have to wait more than a week to attend your nearest session, is crucial: near-instant availability alone makes this one of the most practical therapeutic treatments available. As in Open Dialogue, the secret is equality, the absence of hierarchy and judgement, which leads to solidarity, support and the conviction that the group can together find ways forward for all its members, in ways we simply cannot manage when we are alone.

All of us in that room had two things in common: we had all hit a moment of crisis, and we were all engaged in doing something about it. In the next chapter we look at how crisis comes about, and what happens when it does. Be comforted: crisis drives change. Understood for what they are, crisis and breakdown can be vital, transformative moments. You cannot believe it at the time, but a crisis is the vital first step in recovery. Before you can build a better life, the one you have been living may have to come down.

10. Crisis

A breakdown of any kind is a perfectly normal and understandable reaction to the pressures anyone may find themselves coping with, at any time of life. So if you are helping someone in crisis, the first thing to remember is, this person is not odd or mad or fundamentally different from anyone else. They are not broken. They are not lost. They may be all at sea now, but that is absolutely natural and – strange as it may seem – sensible: their soul, their body or mind has had enough of their situation. They need respite, rest, change and help. And there is an entire world of professionals and systems, overwhelmingly composed of kind and decent and competent people, which exists specifically to help them. A breakdown – whether it takes the form of overwhelming anxiety, self-harm, deep depression or psychosis – is a form of communication.

> **Rule 11: A breakdown is saying, you cannot do this any more; you need to stop and you need to reset. As such, a breakdown is the first step on a journey of healing and recovery. It is NOT a sign that there is anything fundamentally wrong with you.**

Breakdowns of one kind and another are extraordinarily common. They come in many forms – a slow-motion dragging out of a bad time, a burnout, a stage of sleeplessness and worry, a feeling that you are going crazy and cannot cope, an overflowing of unhappiness, or an acute crisis in which you cannot function. One in four of us will have difficulties at some point, according to NHS statistics, but I suspect the statistics are wrong: many more than one in four of my friends and contacts have gone through a really hard time which could be described as a form of breakdown.

We could easily reframe the language; a reset, an adjustment, a correction, a reboot, a transformation, a change, a revision, a shift. People who have been through them, and emerged stronger and happier, have many different ways of seeing breakdown.

Two whom I know saw theirs as 'burnout'. One was unhappy in her relationship, and her job had become too much for her – it was overwhelmingly demanding and unsatisfying, and she felt constantly emotionally and physically exhausted; she was crying a lot, and felt herself creatively blocked. She realised that the elements of life she had come to feel were important – the certainty of a relationship, a job, somewhere to live – were not working for her. She was experiencing certainties as crushing and stultifying. She left her job, broke up with her boyfriend, got another job in another city, reconnected with old friends, then left that second job and that city, deciding, as she put it, 'to become the nomad I have always wanted to be'.

Another, who grew up between the Indian culture of his parents and the British culture in which he was raised, described his breakdown as a 'spiritual emergency'. He found Ayurvedic medicine more useful than Western medication, he says: this three-thousand-year-old system, practised widely throughout India and Nepal, understands health as connection and balance between the body's constitution (*prakriti*) and life forces (*doshas*), part of a system of harmony between the world, the spirit, the body and nature. Through purification, herbal treatments, including oils and spices, yoga and meditation, Ayurveda aims to reduce symptoms, increase resistance to disease, reduce worries and anxieties, and grow feelings of harmony and well-being. While Western medicine treats Ayurveda cautiously, regarding it as complementary therapeutic practice at best, quackery at worst, and in no way a substitute for conventional Western treatments, up to 80 per cent of the population of India use it, either alone or in concert with Western treatments.

Another, who grew up in an Afro-Caribbean home in London, describes a pattern of 'over-resilience' in his background: his family coped with pressure by plunging straight on. Worries, fears and emotions were not discussed, achievement and success were prized, and in the end it became too much for him.

Another, a highly successful professional, coped with relationship breakdown, self-loathing and isolation by taking drugs at home, leading to a spiral of despair and anger. Therapy, anger management and a new relationship wrought a complete change in him.

Another friend found herself crippled by isolation and despair. She took up martial arts and running, and put huge effort into helping her friends, establishing and maintaining a wide and deep network of friends and supporters.

In every case – and I could list dozens more – the lesson is the same: the breakdown happens for clear, unmysterious, logical reasons. Rather than deny or flee it, the wise sufferer accepts and examines those reasons, and finds ways through to a better place.

All this is very well, but when you are in the middle of the storms of a breakdown, the suffering overwhelms the wisdom.

At the first stage of a breakdown, in time of crisis, practical, simple steps are the way forward. So what do you do?

If you sense a crisis approaching, see what you can do to change what you can in your day-to-day routine. Everyone who suffers will feel differently at this stage. For me the warning signs that something is wrong are lowering mood, increasingly negative reactions (I literally hear myself saying 'No' more than 'Yes'); sleep dysregulation (either I stop needing more than five or six hours a night, or I struggle to fall asleep, waking in the small hours and lying there worrying, or I really struggle to get out of bed); increasing anxiety about things I cannot obviously change (the state of the country, the fate of the world, what might happen to me or my loved ones in the future); and then my confidence starts to flag. I begin to feel fearful about doing things that come naturally, normally, like writing or teaching or giving talks; I start to worry unduly and dwell on the normal small reversals of daily life; and then a host of fears follow, about my worth as a parent, as a person, as a writer. The ups and downs of my job, like coming up with good ideas for books, writing them and selling them, start to loom dispropor-tionately. I start to panic about money, about how on earth I will be able to look after my family and myself. In summer I get a different set of warnings: less need of sleep, less caution about plans and spending, overconfi-dence about being able to do it all at the same time, increasing exhaustion, drinking more.

Whatever the change you notice in yourself, this is the moment to tell your employer, your school, your univer-sity, your friends or your family that you are struggling. Do not try to carry on if you feel you cannot carry on. No one knows how the balance between environmental factors and internal pressures is playing out in your case, so your first move is to do what you can to change the environmental ones. Ask yourself, what in my daily life is making me unhappy? What can I do to change? Do I need time off work or study? Do I need to get away for a few days? When was the last time I did something I loved, that made me happy? Can I do that, or something like it, now? Can I make plans, so that I have something to look forward to? What can I do to reduce the pressures I am experiencing from study, work or life?

Do not withdraw into solitary suffering. You need help – so make a fuss. It's nothing to be ashamed of, as we have seen. The pandemic revealed the obvious truth: we all have mental health, so we are all liable to mental ill health. No one is going to think less of you for saying that you need help. God knows, all of us will need help, with one thing or another, at some point in our lives.

Along with talking about it and making any small changes you can, see a doctor before things get out of hand. The Samaritans publish a useful checklist of warning signs.

- Lacking energy or feeling tired
- Feeling exhausted all the time
- Experiencing 'brain fog' (finding it hard to think clearly)
- Finding it hard to concentrate
- Feeling restless and agitated
- Feeling tearful, wanting to cry all the time
- Not wanting to talk to or be with people
- Not wanting to do things you usually enjoy
- Using alcohol or drugs to cope with feelings
- Finding it hard to cope with everyday things and tasks
- Experiencing 'burnout'

If you are experiencing these symptoms, see a doctor. I have come across many people who reach this sort of stage but who fear going to see a GP lest they be designated with a mental health problem and put on drugs. In exactly this state I told my father I was scared of making an appointment in case 'they put me on lithium'. Gently and kindly, my father said, 'No one can make you take anything. Wouldn't it be worth going to see what they say, in case there is something that can help? It can't hurt to go and find out, can it?' He was right, of course.

Whatever happens, by going to a doctor you will have made three vital moves: first, you are now in touch with the services that are there to help you. Second, you have done what for many of us is the hardest thing: you have sought help. Third, and vitally (and it may very well not feel this way), you have started to take power over your suffering. You are now playing the key role in your own recovery – the first step to controlling a condition which might otherwise take control of you.

This is a crucial step for everyone in trouble – and it is especially important for people who are not white and not well-off. For a variety of reasons, the fact is that people living in less wealthy areas and people from black and minority ethnic communities are much less likely to seek and receive help before crises become acute. As a result, first contact with the mental health services is much more likely to come through the police or Accident and Emergency. When in doubt, ask for help.

Clearly, A&E is not the ideal place for someone who is having a mental health crisis, but it is better than the street, or a room filled only with your dangerously despairing thoughts. You can and will receive help, eventually, from an A&E department, so, in an emergency, if you need that help, take it.

If you or someone close to you is in acute crisis, it is time to hit the phone. Depending on your NHS trust, the numbers you are looking for may come up under different headings – Crisis Team, or Intensive Home-Based Treatment Team, Community Mental Health Team, Enhanced Community Mental Health Team, et cetera.

They will be easy to find: search the name of your NHS trust, or your area, and 'mental health crisis support', or call NHS 111, or talk to your GP, or search the internet with the terms 'urgent mental health support' and the name of your area of the country.

Although there is an entire rainforest of different teams with different names offering different services (the NHS is considering employing people to help patients and carers navigate the thousands of 'care pathways' now available), there are broadly two types of in-person help available: Crisis Teams and Community Mental Health Teams. As the names suggest, community teams are there to give long- or short-term care, and support with recovery, while crisis teams offer short-term support.

Whatever they are called, community and crisis teams have a simple purpose: to give the kind of help which keeps you safe, to start you on a road to recovery, and to keep you out of hospital. The idea is, they come to you. The NHS is working towards targets which mean you should be seen by a team within twenty-four hours of referral (and you can self-refer), with urgent cases being seen within four hours.

It can be a strange and unsettling occasion: strangers, professionals, in your room or house or flat, asking questions. When I broke down, my first instinct was to tell the woman who visited me (from a Community Mental Health Team) what I wanted to be true – which was exactly half the truth. I told her I was suffering from seasonal blues (true), in relationship breakdown (true), using cannabis and alcohol (true), but otherwise fine (absolutely not true).

I did not tell her I was barely sleeping, subject to racing thoughts, and careering crazily around, alarming my nearest and dearest. I wish to goodness I had told her the whole truth. What I needed then was a mood stabiliser or antipsychotic, and if I had told her the truth she would have been able to help me make an appointment and obtain a prescription for that medication.

You will experience your own warning signs, depending on what is afflicting you, and depending on how the broad category of your problem plays out in your own individual case. According to the mental health charity Mind, the rates of suffering on any given week in the UK look like this.

- Mixed anxiety and depression: 8 in 100 people
- Generalised anxiety disorder (GAD): 6 in 100 people

- Post-traumatic stress disorder (PTSD): 4 in 100 people
- Depression: 3 in 100 people
- Phobias: 2 in 100 people
- Obsessive-compulsive disorder (OCD): 1 in 100 people
- Panic disorder: fewer than 1 in 100 people

And then there are the conditions which are measured by prevalence over a year or a lifetime.

- Antisocial personality disorder (ASPD): 3 in 100 people (in their lifetime)
- Borderline personality disorder (BPD): 2 in 100 people (in their lifetime)
- Bipolar disorder: 2 in 100 people (in their lifetime)
- Psychotic disorders (including schizophrenia): fewer than 1 in 100 people (in any given year)

(It is worth noting, as Mind does, that these are the terms used in our current treatment models, and that many people find them stigmatising, and reject them for this or other good reasons.)

As you see, by far the most common conditions are in the areas of anxiety and anxiety-depression. If they have come for you, be comforted. You are in wide and wonderful company. Pretty well all of my favourite people, and those I most respect and admire, have experienced anxiety, depression or the exhausting combination of them some call 'burnout'. But do not underestimate them. Anxiety may sound relatively gentle compared to psychosis or schizophrenia, but suffering is not relative; suffering is entirely individual and subjective. Anxiety and depression can be killers, driving suicide, and mutating (if they are not confronted by change, treatment or both) into life-wrecking parasites. The NHS lists the following psychological signs of anxiety which requires action.

- Restlessness
- A sense of dread or fear
- Feeling constantly 'on edge'
- Difficulty concentrating
- Irritability

The NHS advises that:

Your symptoms may cause you to withdraw from social contact [seeing your family and friends] to avoid feelings of worry and dread. You may also find going to work difficult and stressful, and may take time off sick. These actions can make you worry even more about yourself and increase your lack of self-esteem.

Physical symptoms may include:

- dizziness
- tiredness
- a noticeably strong, fast or irregular heartbeat (palpitations)
- muscle aches and tension

- trembling or shaking
- dry mouth
- excessive sweating
- shortness of breath
- stomach ache
- feeling sick
- headache
- pins and needles
- difficulty falling or staying asleep (insomnia).

In the case of my breakdown, I ignored all the warnings and carried on, dodging people who were trying to help me as if they were trying to harm me, telling more half-truths, rising through mania to become more and more ill. Even a weak, unimaginative, categorise-and-prescribe sort of psychiatrist would have made all the difference now. Crisis teams are overseen by psychiatrists who can prescribe quickly. Alas, instead of getting a break and a rest, and having the madness which was growing in me lanced and drained by a few pills, I just got faster, higher, and madder, until I lost contact with reality.

So, when you meet them, tell the community or crisis team the whole truth, and all the details of the truth. Bravery and honesty now can save you from a world of difficulty and distress. As my crack-up continued, I met another member of the team. He came to my flat with a doctor. I felt extremely defensive and fearful that they meant to send for the men in white coats – they *were* the men in white coats, it seemed to me – and so I re-inforced my half-true story, made them cups of tea, did everything I could to hide the other half of the truth and to get them out of the flat, reassured that I did not need them. Two chances for help offered, and two chances thrown away.

The tricky thing at this point is honesty on both sides: be open about what is frightening to you, what you are worried about, what is not working. I now work with intervention teams, training them and briefing them on the sufferer's point of view. Their overwhelming concern is not to commit you to hospital, but to find ways of helping you to be well enough to stay *out* of hospital. There are a series of issues here, and everyone you deal with is going to know them. But even a very honest professional may not necessarily have the time or inclination to share them with you. These issues are:

1. There are not enough psychiatric beds in the country for all those who need them, so there is pressure to keep people out of them, if possible. This can be good – there is less chance you will be forced to have treatment if you do not need it – or not so good, if you really do need it.

2. Some – perhaps many – of the wards where these beds are located are badly run, understaffed, chaotic or scary places, where no one should be treated but many are. The last

few years have seen suicides in the Priory
Hospital Cheadle Royal and at Priory
Woodbourne Hospital, Birmingham; obscene
abuse at Edenfield near Manchester, where
BBC's *Panorama* uncovered an appalling regime
of staff tormenting patients; lethal failings at a
psychiatric hospital run by East London NHS
Foundation Trust, where a patient was able to
inject another with heroin, killing him; and an
ongoing investigation into mental health deaths
in NHS trusts across Essex.

In 2019, I interviewed a former patient at the
Broadoak Unit in Broadgreen Hospital,
Liverpool, who described revolting
mistreatment by staff and security contractors.
Six people were suspended from that unit in
2016, but a former patient who now visits
hospitals as an expert patient and survivor
researcher at psychiatric units told me that they
have seen and heard evidence that
incompetence, abuse and inadequate care
continue to plague psychiatric wards across the
country.

There is no clear picture, nationally, of
which wards are good and which are failing.
People in the system – and these are often
wonderful people, who have dedicated their
professional lives to helping the mentally
ill – know about the bad ones, but they despair

that anything will be done to change them. For example, I recently took part in a training session for Approved Mental Health Professionals (the social workers who have the power to detain you under the Mental Health Act) from a Welsh NHS trust where one attendee said the worst part of his job comes after an assessment, when he is sure that someone needs care and he has made out the detention order, 'And then they say, "There's a bed available in Unit X," and your heart just sinks, because you know that it's the worst possible place for someone in distress.'

3. There are worries among psychiatrists that because too many people are being committed to hospital, a system of 'gatekeeping' has sprung up, which is designed to keep people out of wards, and which rejects people who need treatment. One practising psychiatrist, who was herself treated in a psychiatric unit for a severe eating disorder, told me that she was extremely careful to be a 'good patient', to do nothing to challenge or inconvenience the staff, to fit neatly into a diagnostic category and to cooperate with the treatment the staff wanted to give, rather than demand anything different that she felt she might need. The danger, she said, was that she might be given a diagnosis of borderline personality disorder as

a punishment, as a way of saying, 'We can't help you, go away,' and thus be excluded from care.

4. Pressures on services and concern that too many people are being detained under the Mental Health Act mean that the criteria for access to a bed for acute crisis are being made more rigorous. At the time of writing people can be detained for their 'own health or safety or with a view to the protection of other persons'. But researchers, NHS directors and policymakers are proposing that this will change to 'there is a substantial likelihood of significant harm to the health, safety or welfare of the person, or the safety of any other person'.

Conclusion: if you are friend or family to someone who is in acute crisis, and you are sure they need to be treated in hospital without delay, you cannot be half-hearted in what you say about their case. Going through the minds of the crisis team, the doctor and the social worker who will make out the order to detain (as described above, this person is called an AMHP, an Approved Mental Health Professional) will be this phrase: '*substantial likelihood of significant harm to self or others . . .*'

If you need to get them into hospital, then this is what you need to say. The chances are that this *is* your reasoning, so make it very clear.

Most people who are detained in a psychiatric bed are judged to be a risk to themselves, rather than others. If you think this is true of you or someone close to you, be categorical about it.

> **Rule 12: If you are certain that someone you care about needs help, and you find yourself fighting to get it for them, use the most forceful and unambiguous language: fight in the terms the system understands.**

If you want the services you need to stop minimising the problem or excluding the sufferer from care, say this: 'I wish it to be put on record that I believe there is a substantial likelihood of significant harm to this person, and I am keeping a record of this conversation, and you can be sure the coroner will hear of it if you deny them the care they need.'

In the case of hospitalisation, what happens next is dealt with in Chapter 16 'On the ward'. But let us pull back a bit and examine what happens in the happier case, when the Crisis Team / Home-Based Treatment Team / AMHP are able to keep the sufferer out of hospital, and begin their care, treatment and healing at home.

There is no typical crisis team worker – the one thing that characterises good people throughout the system is a particular gentleness, which is remarkable and common and widespread and unmistakeable. It's a gentleness in the eyes, a seeking to understand, a sort of listening look. You will know it when you see it. If you do not see it, if you see a kind of brusqueness, a shutters-down kind of impatience, steer well clear. If you get shutters-down treatment from a shutters-down type – or if you fear that someone you are helping is getting that – then get ready to make a loud complaint and a hell of a fuss. In my experience you are much more likely to find this in in-patient settings where chaotic environments, understaffing, poor supervision and poor leadership have led to toxic teams and abuse scandals of the kinds listed above. (See also Chapter 16.)

Let us put people and practices to all this information. In a field which is rich in caring and thoughtful people, an inspiring example is Tamara Moon, an assistant practitioner on a crisis team. Having graduated with a BSc in psychology she worked at Crisis Point in Manchester, a residential short-term service, a kind of third way between care at home and care in hospital. She moved to London where she now works on a team in Islington, an inner-city borough with a population of a quarter of a million. Her story is illustrative because she is an example of the current generation of young people coming into the sector, the practitioners who staff the front line, the kind you are most likely to meet, and who will be the leaders of tomorrow. Currently one of the most junior members of the team, she spends a great deal of time at the sharp end, with people who need help. Her job is to go out to homes and flats all over the borough to assist people in every kind of trouble. Listening is fundamental to her role – listening to distress and being a sounding board: someone who aims to sympathetically and dispassionately untangle what is happening to the person in trouble, and offer ways through.

Her first concern is safety: are you safe, now, and is she safe with you? She will ask you about your living conditions, while making her own observations. Is this a sanitary environment? Are you managing to care for yourself: to feed, clothe, wash and care for yourself? Now she wants to know about your daily life. Do you have a routine? Who do you see? Who do you talk to? The point is to establish what she can about your networks and relationships. As Tamara says, no one knows more about what is happening to a person in trouble than they do – and those closest to them. This can be a most rewarding and heartening part of the conversation.

'One of my favourite parts of the job is the networks that people are part of, the families that are around them, the people in the community,' Tamara told me. 'I had an experience recently; I was in a lady's home and her neighbour came upstairs and I do think that she'd been completely unaware of how much the lady who lived above her was struggling. There was a look of complete and utter care and compassion in her face. And she embraced her. And it just looked like the forging of a new support system right there, happening in front of me. It was just really amazing.'

The conversation will go on to cover your symptoms.

Are you sleeping? How are you feeling? Are you using drugs and/or alcohol? What has happened to you and is happening that is making you unhappy? How does that unhappiness manifest in your feelings and doings?

The next stage is to make a plan for your well-being, either informally, which means talking through steps you can take to improve your situation, or more formally, which means a Care Plan.

A Care Plan is intended to be a clear and logical series of needs and steps covering your situation, what might happen, and what should. It is drawn up by a social worker, an Approved Mental Health Professional on the Crisis Team. Templates vary, but the basic format is a list of your identified needs down the left-hand side of the page, a column in the middle with interventions, and a column on the right with aims and outcomes.

'Identified needs' describes your situation, what has happened to you, the history of what you have been feeling and how it affected you, when and why. So, for example: 'In January, Jones began experiencing depression due to stress / life events. Since February, Jones has felt unable to go to work, they have been experiencing relationship difficulties with their partner, and have been experiencing feelings of severely low mood and thoughts and incidents of self-harm. As a result Jones is in a situation of serious vulnerability. Jones has been using alcohol, which they feel has had a negative effect on their ability to function and self-care, and on their relationship. Jones says they want to reduce or stop drinking, which they believe is a trigger for deterioration in their mental health. Jones expresses serious concern that they may self-harm, and they are keen to access support and psychological services to alleviate their depression.'

This is only a short example: the Identified Needs section of a Care Plan should be a detailed, accurate and thoughtful record and assessment of your situation, running to hundreds of words.

The 'Interventions' column details the course of action you and the practitioner will come up with between you, taking into account any access to doctors, psychiatrists or services you have had or may need.

So, in our example: 'Jones has been allocated a care coordinator from the Community Mental Health Team who will maintain contact with them with a view to monitoring their mental health and providing support in relation to this as required. They have indicated that they are happy for their care coordinator to liaise with their partner if there are concerns about their mental health. They have been prescribed [an antidepressant]. They have concerns about side effects and the length of the treatment, and it is important that they are able to discuss this with relevant medical professionals. Their medication in the community will be reviewed by Dr Smith. Jones has been referred to Recovery Steps Drug and Alcohol services and registered for eight appointments with a Psychological Well-Being Practitioner [therapist].'

The 'Aims/Outcomes' column is fairly bland. So, for example: 'To promote stability in Jones's mental health, to avoid self-harm, to reduce use of alcohol, and for additional support to be offered quickly if there are signs of deterioration.' But it is good to agree what the goals are, and important to establish what steps will be taken if they are missed.

Lower down, the Care Plan becomes more interesting. First there is the 'Contingency Plan', which details steps to be taken if Jones fails to turn up to an appointment with Dr Smith, for example, or misses appointments with the therapist or the Crisis Team. The steps tend to be: telephone Jones, contact GP, contact nominated carer (Jones's partner), visit Jones.

Next comes 'Relapse Indicators / Initial Interventions'. In Jones's case this might be: 'Increased use of alcohol, deepening depression, increased incidence of thoughts of self-harm, or self-harm.'

It is followed by 'Crisis Plan'. In our example this would read along the lines of: 'Increased support from Community Mental Health Team including medication review. Liaise with Jones's partner. Consider referral to the Home-Based Treatment Team with hospital admission being considered as a last resort.'

If you are offered a Care Plan, make sure you are happy with every aspect of it before signing it off. Pay particular attention to the 'Interventions' column if there are boxes marked 'No intervention entered'. This is where you will find the services trying to balance your needs with their ability to provide. If Jones is self-harming, is it sufficient that they have been referred to a

Psychological Well-Being Practitioner for eight online appointments? When are these going to take place? Does Jones actually need regular visits from the Home-Based Treatment Team? Is there a date for the review of medication with Dr Smith? Does Jones have a date for their first appointment with the Steps alcohol service? Are there other addiction and drug use services Jones should know about?

All this sounds very bureaucratic and theoretical (though there is every reason to expect that Jones, given the kind of support their Care Plan calls for, will begin to recover rapidly); the real nub of the issue is how much help and support we can get when we need it, and how skilfully it is delivered.

Nothing beats caring and expert human contact, so it is time to consider a third way, between treatment at home and hospital – a crisis house. Some are run by the NHS, some are run by charities and independent bodies, and others in partnership. They offer short-term residential support to help manage a really hard time: if you are not feeling safe at home, or if your environment is unbearable or making you worse, if you need close help and support, a crisis house can be a life-changer.

Tamara Moon worked at such a place: Crisis Point in Manchester. She told me how it functions.

Crisis Point is a short-term residential service. So somebody might come in and spend perhaps a week there. And often the circumstances, the environment that somebody has come from, the environment where the crisis has taken place essentially, is enough to maintain it. So you take somebody out of that environment where they are physically at risk of harm, and give them somewhere where all of their basic needs are catered for, there's food available, it's warm, and they've got professionals around them, many of whom aren't from a medical background [as well as nurses and doctors] but are just there because they care. And then we listen and make suggestions and just spend time with them. The difference that we see in people is really, really incredible. We do this through lots of activities. I've never played so much pool in my life! And lots of card games. We had a pool table and actually I found that it was on night shifts that somebody is most likely to tell you all of these really distressing, difficult thoughts they've been having. They would open up about really difficult experiences and maybe speak about their goals and what they want to be different. The time that someone's most honest is when everybody else has gone. You know, all the nurses, the doctors have gone home. There's less noise. The lights are dimmed. You're playing a game of cards. Those are the times that somebody is more likely to open up. And actually, in my experience, that's where the magic happens.

Tamara showed me around the low nondescript building on the northern edge of central Manchester. There was nothing on the outside to indicate that this was a place where magic happens: a square of tarmac, a table and chairs, a scrappy buddleia bush. Inside, a warm day room, a pool table, small bookshelves, a TV and sofas, comfy chairs, and doors to bedrooms and a kitchen leading off. A middle-aged man looked up from scrolling through his phone and said hello. It takes so little, you realise, to make people feel safe. Nothing spectacular, nothing especially beautiful, no views (at least from the day room); just an atmosphere of calm, of company. Below, behind and beyond all the interventions we use to help people in crisis or in suffering, beyond medication, therapy, changes in lifestyle and behaviour, beyond the mighty remedies of that trinity of recovery – nature, activity and purpose – is the most powerful of all: gentle and sympathetic human contact.

At their best, crisis houses work this way. To be in the quiet hours with someone like Tamara – who will sit and listen, draw you out with empathy and understanding, patience and concern – must be to experience a great lifting of the world's weight from you. Again, the statistics which say one in four of us would benefit greatly from this kind of contact – will need it, at some point – are almost certainly a great underestimation. I do not know anyone who has not struggled, who does not struggle. Most strikingly, it is many of these people, who work in the mental health system having suffered, or who continue to suffer, who are among its most effective members. From support workers to consultants, via mental health nurses, Approved Mental Health Professionals, via GPs, mental health pharmacists, members of home-based treatment teams, members of crisis teams and police officers, there is a large (though uncounted) population of people who know mental health from the inside, who are responsible for operating and administering it. They give the lie to the idea that 'we' who may have had or do have or will have problems are different from 'them', the 'normal' ones, those who 'don't have mental health issues'. In the 1950s the introduction of chlorpromazine (marketed under the brand names of Thorazine and Largactil among others) changed psychiatric treatment dramatically, giving hundreds of thousands of people relief from acute psychotic symptoms over the decades since. In our time, perhaps the most beneficial conceptual leap in psychotherapy and in the public conception of mental health is the idea of the spectrum – and the notion that we are all on an arc which stretches from very well to very ill, and that, depending on our histories and circumstances, we can all move along it in either direction.

> **Rule 13: The idea that 'they', the 'normal', are over there, in their great successful majority, and that 'we', the sufferers, are over here, in our particular personal torment, is an illusion.**

When I was ill and under section, a support worker took me to the café which served the hospital, beyond the locked ward. What was most moving and most therapeutic was listening to his story, how he had flown high in work in London, and broken down, and come North, and found himself looking after people. The half-hour in the café, the cheap tea and the view of the car park, were my crisis house. They come in other forms – in drop-in centres, refuges, safe spaces. You might find them in a friend's living room or through your NHS Talking Therapies / IAPT service. Mind and Rethink Mental Illness list them and ways of finding them on their websites – Mind's is particularly good.

At the time of writing a shift towards halfway houses, drop-in centres and so-called 'crisis cafés' is taking place. It springs from a desire to take the police out of their significant role in attending mental health crises and replace them with specialist responders. So, the plan goes, the car that turns up at your house will be branded NHS rather than POLICE, and will be crewed by professional mental health workers with the means to medicate you, rather than officers with the means to cuff you.

Some regions of England and Wales record police attending up to 80 per cent of mental health incidents. Police leaders and politicians are planning to reduce this to 20 per cent, with officers attending only when there is a threat to life. Plans to manage this transition include a nationwide network of twenty-four-hour mental health helplines, specialist mental health ambulances and, notably, a proposed £1 billion investment in community mental health services. Expect to see more crisis cafés and, hopefully, crisis houses like the Crisis Point centre described above. While crisis houses are run in individual ways and offer different services, the basics are overnight accommodation for a limited time (a week or two); small numbers of beds; a safe, home-like environment; and expert staff on hand to help. Crisis cafés are drop-in centres characterised by a supportive and non-judgemental atmosphere. They tend to be run by calm staff who see and help a great many people in trouble simply by taking an understanding and sympathetic approach, and having information on all the relevant support services and treatment options in the local area. Visiting one in North Liverpool (I was researching and interviewing, rather than in need, at the time), I found a quiet and gentle place which felt like a cross between a library and a café, full of information about local support networks, interest and hobby groups, staffed by people who were able to offer information and advice. I would recommend such places to anyone: even getting myself together to leave the house and go to the crisis café, have a cup of tea and read a leaflet would have been a step in the right direction when I was down in the misery pit. I would have been doing something to take control of my condition and my own destiny, howsoever small.

11. Medication: Background and basics

The great breakthrough in psychiatric medication came in the 1950s, with chlorpromazine, intended as an anaesthetic until a French naval surgeon named Henri Laborit began giving it to injured soldiers as a treatment for shock. Laborit observed that it reduced hyper-vigilance, panic and distress. He noted a numbing effect: people taking the drug showed less interest in their surroundings. Induced apathy and indifference may not sound exactly desirable, but for Laborit and pioneering French psychiatrists treating mania, psychosis and schizophrenia, these effects were seen and felt to be miraculous. Chlorpromazine vanquished hallucinations, delusions and mania. Marketed as Thorazine, chlorpromazine was given to two million patients in the US alone within eight months of its introduction. Schizophrenia had suddenly become a treatable disease. People who had been in acute distress achieved remission in weeks. Modern psychiatry had begun.

Huge numbers of sufferers were discharged from mental institutions: in the US the hospitalised population fell from half a million to fewer than 200,000. This was not an unalloyed good – care in the community is all very well if there is care and a community available, which for many sufferers, there wasn't, and still isn't – but chlorpromazine created the era in which we now live: the psychiatrist as a medication-dispensing medical doctor, prescribing drugs which have powerful beneficial effects on the symptoms at which they are targeted, and, in many cases, strikingly negative side effects on the body and brain.

Heinz Lehmann, who introduced chlorpromazine to the US, and was astounded by its power to free people from the symptoms of schizophrenia, described the side effects as the equivalent of a 'chemical lobotomy'. And here is the crux of the medication question: the balance between the life-changing good it can do you, and the negative consequences of medication's side effects.

Although there has been no breakthrough of a similar magnitude in the decades since the creation of chlorpromazine, many hundreds of different drugs have been developed. Psychiatrists and doctors now prescribe medication for anxiety and eating disorders, depression, psychosis and schizophrenia, borderline personality disorder, et cetera: there is not a mental health condition for which a psychiatrist cannot suggest a drug which could help. This chapter is for you if you or someone you care for is taking or thinking about taking medication. None of it is my conjecture or opinion: as you will see, the following information is based on research by and interviews with expert professionals. My findings reveal that there are some fundamental points to consider about taking medication, and several useful ways of approaching the subject.

*

As we have seen in Chapter 5, there are no biomarkers for your troubles. For most common conditions, your psychiatrist or doctor is unable to look at a scan of your brain, mind, body or soul and see something wrong with you. Instead, you are understood and treated by your symptoms – by how you feel and act, and by how you describe how you feel and act.

Although it would be convenient and helpful if we could detect an imbalance in your brain chemicals, the idea of a chemical imbalance remains a hypothesis – an unproven theory. This may be reassuring (we don't know if there is anything 'wrong' with your brain) or it may not – something is obviously wrong, and we need to do something about it.

It would be wonderful if we knew exactly how psychiatric drugs work, but the truth is we do not. Professional and academic thinking suggests, for example, that many antidepressants *may* work by increasing levels of serotonin in the brain, which makes us feel happier. However, recent professional and academic studies have questioned this. A review by researchers at University College London published in the journal *Molecular Psychiatry* in 2023 examined findings on the relationship between serotonin and depression in tens of thousands of people. The review was a meta-study, a study of clinical and academic studies, rather than a clinical investigation in its own right. Some psychiatrists criticised its findings on that basis, but meta-studies are the means by which researchers gain the broadest understanding of a given field. One finding, widely reported in the international media, was that comparisons of levels of serotonin in the blood and brain do not reveal differences between people with depression and those without.

When serotonin levels are artificially lowered in hundreds of healthy volunteers, the study found, they did not become depressed.

The report's lead author, Joanna Moncrieff, is a psychiatrist who has published and spoken regularly and prolifically on her scepticism about the prevalence of drug treatments like antidepressants and lithium. She believes that we are prescribing too widely, and giving people false information about the relationship between neurotransmitters, chemicals and how we feel. She points to studies showing that the more stress we experience, the more likely we are to meet depression. 'Our view is that patients should not be told that depression is caused by low serotonin or by a chemical imbalance, and they should not be led to believe that antidepressants work by targeting these unproven abnormalities,' Moncrieff has said. She and other researchers point out that it is possible that antidepressants work by an enhanced placebo effect, or by blunting emotions in general.

This study was soon answered and contradicted by another, from an equally respected institution, Imperial College London. Using a brain-imaging scanner, researchers found that serotonin release as a response to amphetamines (known to increase serotonin) was lower in 17 depressed patients than it was in 12 healthy volunteers.

It is worth noting that mainstream psychiatry vehemently rejects the position held by researchers like Joanna Moncrieff, while accepting that she and those who agree with her are dedicated and expert professionals who, like all the best people in the field, are motivated by finding better ways to help people. They worry that if you believe you are feeling low because there is an imbalance in your brain chemicals, you may feel pessimistic about your chances of changing your feelings without chemical help. You may feel condemned to depression, and lack faith in your ability to feel better without antidepressants, in which case you may come to rely on antidepressants.

It is also worth knowing that it is not disputed that 20 to 30 per cent of patients do not respond to the most common class of antidepressants, selective serotonin reuptake inhibitors: we do not know why, but the drugs simply do not help this group.

Do not panic. There are sensible and helpful ways through all this.

The first thing to understand is that when it comes to medication, you and your clinician are embarked on a joint project, which is to find the correct medication for you, which you can take for the shortest possible time in the lowest effective dosage to the best possible effect.

The second thing to understand is that the lowest effective dosage for you *may* be zero.

I visited a laboratory in Oxford where they are

working on antidepressants for children and young people. Professor Catherine Harmer, a leading researcher in the field, showed me some brain scans made by an MRI scanner, which displayed areas of the brain in which you could see enhanced activity (measured by levels of oxygen) after the subject had taken antidepressants. I was surprised by how large was the scale: we were not looking at neurons and serotonin molecules; we were looking at a wide and unsubtle outline of the brain, which showed that the prefrontal cortex – a part of the brain involved in planning, working memory and decision-making – was busy, judging by the levels of oxygen it was getting through. When I am miserable I struggle with all these things – according to the serotonin hypothesis, low levels of serotonin are interfering with these functions. According to the same theory, if you are able to take drugs which boost the level, you boost mood and, in turn, functionality. Professor Harmer, a highly respected professional at a prestigious institution, whose career and research funding are thoroughly bound up in the development of antidepressants, said something unforgettable. I asked if she would take antidepressants; if she would give them to her children.

'Yes,' she said. 'If I'd tried absolutely everything else.'

It is worth pausing over this. Someone who knows as much as anyone about what these pills do and how they might work, who is paid and employed to expand their efficacy and use, would use them in the last resort.

So when it comes to the most common kind of

psychiatric drugs – antidepressants prescribed for depression or anxiety – (we are not talking about psychosis, mania, loss of touch with reality or full-on breakdown here, all of which can be hugely helped immediately with antipsychotic medication, but rather about the much more common conditions of anxiety and depression), the third thing to understand is this:

Rule 14: If nothing else works, if you really have tried everything else, if you are in need of a last resort, then that is what medication is there for.

As must be clear by now, we are in the realms of trial and error and anecdote and what works for you. There is no exact science here, but there are lots of choices and paths to explore.

One friend has taken the antidepressant citalopram for a long time. He says he does not know if he needs it now, though he felt he did when he started taking it; he does not know how or if it works; it may be that he feels better because of a placebo effect – and none of this matters to him, because he is able to live a happy and productive life.

Another friend was in a period of low mood and misery and preparing to go to the doctor to get a prescription for antidepressants. But before she took that step, she decided to try other things. She went swimming. She took regular walks. She trained as a yoga teacher. She started a business. She began to see a therapist. She found she did not need antidepressants after all.

Another, suffering from chronic fatigue and feelings of helplessness and hopelessness, obtained an appointment with a psychiatrist. He asked after her symptoms, which included feelings of wanting to end it all. He asked her repeatedly whether her joints hurt, and whether she could touch her toes: a similar condition to hers, fibromyalgia, causes pain in the joints and all over the body. She told him her joints were fine; she had no physical pain. He prescribed sertraline, a common antidepressant. He made no follow-up appointment – he wrote her a prescription and dismissed her. She took the sertraline, which helped, arresting her lowest moods, and after six months stopped taking it. In that time she had no contact from the psychiatrist or the surgery: nothing. She was left to manage the antidepressants and her condition entirely by herself.

During the pandemic, a friend went through lockdown in a basement flat. He was unable to work, he saw few people and he became terribly miserable. Any doctor who had seen him then would have prescribed antidepressants. But then lockdown ended, he went back to work and began a new relationship. No antidepressant could have wrought the wonderful change which came over his state of mind and his feelings.

A young student in his final year at school found he was miserable and anxious, and in a relationship that was making him unhappy. He went to a doctor who prescribed antidepressants. The student began taking them – because he was over eighteen his parents were

not told. When his father found packets of the medication, the boy told him he had taken them for a couple of
weeks, and not liked the side effects, and come off. He
had not consulted the doctor about stopping – he just
stopped. His exams came and he did well; he went to
university where he met someone wonderful and began
a fulfilling relationship.

There are as many experiences of medications as
there are people taking them, but there are some lessons
we can draw from the examples above: you might not
need them; they might help; you may receive very little
help with choosing or managing them; you may find
yourself making decisions about stopping or tapering
usage which should be made by a clinician; unless you
are in a manic or psychotic state, no one is going to be
more expert in their effects, for good and ill, than you. In
a mist of maybes and perhapses, what we need is the
greatest possible certainty.

Assuming you are in a position where medication is or
might be right for you, here are some points to bear in
mind.

The conversation you have with your clinician now
will set the course for what follows, so it is worth taking
real time over it. Do not be rushed.

Dr Swapnil Gupta, Associate Professor and Medical
Director of Ambulatory Psychiatry at Mount Sinai
Morningside Hospital, New York, is an authority on de-
prescribing, on taking people off pills, not because she is

against medication but because she is against over-medication. As she tells Angie Peacock in an excellent interview for Angie's series of conversations about mental health on her YouTube channel, Professor Gupta trained in India, where many patients paid for their treatments out of their own pockets. In India, she says, treatment is strictly evidence-based, and this combination of necessity and normal local practice (one kind of drug at a time) meant that most of her patients were taking only one drug. Moving to practise in America, she was amazed to find it was common for people to take several at once.

'There really is no evidence base for such gross poly-pharmacy, for six to eight drugs at a time,' she says. Britain and Europe are ahead of the US in this regard: poly-pharmacy is less common here, but it is still an issue. Professor Gupta has had a great deal of success reducing people's doses to the minimum, and here is her advice, as given to Angie Peacock, quoted here with her permission, and a rule to remember:

Rule 15: If you are offered a medication, always ask why you are being offered it. Ask what else you could take instead of this, i.e. why this one, why now?

Ask if there are ways to manage what you are feeling without taking medication. What are those ways? What can you do?

Next, and vitally, Professor Gupta advises that you

ask about checking your progress: 'When will we meet to re-evaluate the necessity of this medicine, and its effects?'

Do not be fobbed off with a vague appointment sometime in the future: get a date.

It is never too early to talk about stopping or discontinuing. Professor Gupta believes it should be part of the first conversation: 'How long shall I take this for before we look at tapering off?'

Many clinicians have serious concerns about the automatic renewal of prescriptions without regular and detailed evaluation of the medication's effects. I have come across the same thing: a young man who had a breakdown went to see his doctor about reducing his dosage of a mood stabiliser. The doctor refused to have the conversation, wrote him an identical prescription for more of the same, and sent him on his way. The young man really wanted to taper his dose down to a minimum with a view to coming off, but the clinician gave him no help, no support and no impression that such a course might be possible. This goes against all the values of clinical practice: if you find yourself in this position, object in the strongest possible terms, demand a second opinion, or a different doctor, and be prepared to make a complaint. The evidence shows that making a fuss gets you the best treatment. If necessary, make that fuss.

The background here is that your clinician may have clear ideas about what could and should be best for you, based on what has worked for people with similar presentations, but your clinician does not *know*. Thus your clinician may set about trying to find out what is right for you by prescribing according to trial and error. Effectively, you are both performing an experiment in which your well-being is the subject. You may be advised to take a certain dose, wait for it to work, and then monitor how you feel, and any side effects, and report back, either for a change of pill, or for another to offset side effects, or for a different dose, or a combination of these.

Always remember, what is important is not the clinician's time, or the pressures on the system, or what has worked for other people. All that matters is what is right for you. As Professor Gupta puts it, 'If your questions are met with anger or defensiveness on the part of the provider, it's the fault of the provider.'

Of course we all want to help our doctors, and we are extremely sympathetic to beleaguered health systems, but there is a time to be a biddable and obedient patient, and there is a time to put your foot down. Taking psychiatric medication of any kind is emphatically the latter.

Another point to be aware of is that word of mouth and the wormholes of the internet mean that many people arrive in surgeries wanting and expecting to be given medication. 'Physicians in their practices face a lot of pressure,' Dr Gupta says. 'It's an age of quick fixes. The patient is coming in saying, "I want to get rid of my depression." The doctor thinks the way to do this is a pill. Both the patient and the doctor are enlisted in the same delusion – a pill is going to fix the problem.'

The inference is important: medication addresses symptoms, not causes.

Dr Gupta continues, 'Patients feel very attracted to a medicine even before they come to clinic, so I experience a lot of pressure from my patients to prescribe certain medications, and I try my best to resist that pressure.'

If you meet a clinician like Dr Gupta, whose first step is to investigate if there are ways other than medication for you to address the way you feel, then fortune is with you. Remember Professor Harmer, Oxford researcher, above: '*If I'd tried absolutely everything else.*'

If you meet a clinician who thinks that medication may be the best way forward for you, then the questions, the care to establish how little you need to take and for how short a time you need to take it, and when you will meet again to discuss it, will likely come from you.

A crucial point here is to listen to what your clinician says about how long the medication will take to work. Psychiatrists agonise over this: they prescribe a medication that they know has beneficial effects, but they also know – and tell their patients – that it does not work immediately. The patient takes the pill but it seems to do nothing: waking up the next day, and the day after, and the day after that with no apparent change causes double distress. The pills don't seem to be working and the patient is in exactly the same miserable, distressed or dangerous emotional place they were when they first sought help. So if you are told a medication takes a while to work, you can and must trust that this is true.

It is worth taking real trouble over medication because it is an uncertain subject, even among clinicians who dispense medication every day. The reasons for this are various and fascinating in themselves. Drug trials are overwhelmingly funded by the pharmaceutical companies who make and market the drugs, so everyone involved has an interest in declaring them effective and safe. Multiple independent studies show that many drugs are only marginally more effective than placebos, if at all. For example, paroxetine, a common antidepressant marketed as Seroxat or Paxil, was studied by a group of psychiatrists on behalf of the World Health Organisation, who compared it to placebos. They concluded that this popular drug was 'not superior to placebo in terms of overall treatment effectiveness'. This does not mean it will not work for you – it just means that if you believe that something else you are taking (like a placebo) will work for you, it is just as likely to do so as paroxetine. It is worth keeping in mind that it actually does not matter why a drug works, or if it is actually any better than a placebo. If it works, it works. And if your pill is not working for you it does not mean you have a treatment-resistant condition. In a great many cases, medication which works for one patient does not work for another.

When you are talking to your clinician, consider the pressures on him, her or them, too. They want to help you; they do not know how beneficial or harmful medication will be for you (since no one reacts to a given medication in quite the same way as anyone else) and they may lack all the powers they would wish to send to your aid: they will not be in a position to send you to an advanced research lab, or scan your brain, or make repeat appointments in order to monitor you closely. And they will surely hesitate to make some of the recommendations which may cross their mind while addressing your case. The solution to what is making you miserable, for example, might be, 'Leave your relationship, which clearly is not working; change the job/course which is making you unhappy; eat five portions of fresh fruit and vegetables every day; get at least eight hours' sleep every night; go swimming or running three times a week; take up yoga/kickboxing/Qi-gong/volunteering in your community: I guarantee you will feel ten times better by this time next month.' But although an enlightened physician might well advocate these kinds of changes, many others may feel this kind of social prescribing is beyond their scope, and so they default to medication.

When I have worked with and talked to psychiatrists they have told me that they hesitate, often, to act in ways which their peers might judge 'radical'. Radical may be a term of admiration in art and literature. In psychiatry it is not. Fall ill in Belgium, however, as one of my correspondents did, and you may find yourself with a prescription for trips to art galleries and good places to see blossom and take walks in the woods.

Whether or not you decide to take medication, bear in mind this point, made by Professor Mike Slade of the

University of Nottingham, an international authority on recovery and mental health, in his book *Personal Recovery and Mental Illness*:

> Overall, a balanced appraisal of the effectiveness of medication would be that medication has some benefits, generally modest, for some people some of the time. David Whitwell – a practising psychiatrist – asks an important question: 'If only 50% derive benefit from the drugs, why are 100% still being encouraged to take them? The 50% who do not benefit may be positively disadvantaged by the unwanted effects of the drug. Efforts to raise the amount that patients actually take of the prescribed drugs fail to address well-founded patient scepticism.'

Professor Slade goes on to cite a famous study, the Vermont longitudinal study, which followed 118 patients, diagnosed as severely ill, over 32 years. The results for those who were judged to be recovered were remarkable.

> 20% were prescribed no psychotropic medication; 30% were prescribed but did not take any medication; 25% were prescribed and made targeted use; 25% were prescribed and 'religiously' took their medication.

His conclusion is heartening and deeply helpful: I feel it should be borne in mind by anyone who considers, takes or decides not to take psychiatric medication (the emphasis is mine).

Some patients will take medication as suggested by the prescriber. Some will negotiate the dose, type or duration of prescription. Some will choose non-pharmacological approaches to self-management. *All choices are valid, because making choices promotes self-determination and personal responsibility.*

For what it is worth, my own approach to medication is twofold. In time of crisis I found it absolutely invaluable. I did not enjoy taking quetiapine but I am tremendously glad I did. It was as dramatic as the accounts of the effects of chlorpromazine on severely ill patients with which we began this chapter – I was in awful distress, as mad as a snake, before I took it. Sixty hours and two large doses later, I was back: shaky, uncertain, with a lot to process and a long recovery ahead. But back: sane and returning to stability.

In the years since, when in hard times, I have taken the advice of an eminent psychiatrist who told me, 'Don't go to bad doctors, don't go to poor psychiatrists, don't take medication if you don't need it. Your condition is clearly seasonal, so use light therapy and if you can't sleep, take tryptophan.' (Tryptophan is a sleep support and a mild antidepressant, available without prescription. I have used it for a couple of weeks during my most taxing time of year, which falls somewhere between mid-November and early January.)

Most people I know who live productive lives alongside their struggles with well-being (which go beyond the kind that everyone experiences) work in a similar way: they take a carefully personalised approach, choosing to be cautious towards medication, but unafraid to try it when it seems necessary.

12. Medication: Practicalities, according to an expert

Meet Juliet Shepherd. Juliet has over twenty-two years' professional experience of psychiatric medication: she is a former president of the College of Mental Health Pharmacy and a sunny, unafraid, deeply caring person, currently the Senior Pharmacist at the Herefordshire and Worcestershire Health and Care NHS Trust. I asked her about how she understands and works with mental health medication. From the outset, her answers took me by surprise.

'Medication is usually a stepping stone towards the next step in life,' Juliet began. 'So it helps people to get to do the things they wanted to do. It's not the *answer*. You know, you can sit at home with depression and then you can sit at home taking an antidepressant with depression that's not changed your life. Now you've got side effects. So the next bit is the hard work. Taking the tablet is relatively simple – the hard work happens when you have to walk out the front door again.'

'If you were prescribed antidepressants,' I ask, 'how would you feel about it?'

'I'd do it,' she says, immediately. 'I would definitely take it, and I'm not very good at taking medication.'

I press her. 'A lot of young people are resistant to

taking antidepressants because they've heard bad stories. Cath Harmer said, "*If I'd tried absolutely everything else.*" It sounded as though medication really should be the last resort?'

Juliet nods. 'Yes, definitely. Antidepressants are about step three or step four. It does depend. There are people I have seen with whom it will be step number one, because when you hear them talking you're scared they're going to take their own life. And it may look like we've jumped to step four. I'm not going to sit there and ask them if they're going out for regular walks, because that isn't acceptable. And if I read *another thing* about Parkrun [free weekly running events organised by volunteers and attended by people around the world] keeping everybody healthy, I might just shoot someone. It undermines somebody with severe depression. Going for a run isn't going to do it – can they get up and clean their teeth? With depression especially, there's a wide range of understanding and [a wide range] of the illness itself. People are getting better at that, at looking at that spectrum and saying, "I'm probably now halfway down the spectrum of how ill I am," or, "Actually, yes, I'm just fed up today, and getting outside and doing something will make me feel better."'

'Would you worry about side effects? About coming off it?' I ask.

Juliet grins. 'I do a workshop when I'm training staff: I give people a list of the side effects that might come with a medication. I ask them to get together and work out which is the worst side effect. And then I watch them all having a massive argument about whether weight gain or constipation is the worst thing that you've ever had. And obviously what you'll discover is that everybody is different. For example, I've never had constipation in my life so it wouldn't bother me – I think it might be quite a relief at times – and then for other people, you know, weight gain would be the absolute thing they couldn't manage. So it depends.

'Personally, I would try to be as open as possible with the person that had prescribed to me. Especially if I was getting a side effect that I couldn't manage or felt like I couldn't manage *no matter how embarrassing it is*. Because there are side effects that happen with these medications that the British people will not want to talk about, constipation being one of them.

'So I would try to make an effort to be as open as possible, because there might be something that could have been done about it. But being a British stoical person, which is my natural way of being, might mean I stopped taking that tablet because I couldn't bear it any longer. You could write a whole chapter about STOP BEING BRITISH! That would be useful.'

So, with that in mind, here's my next rule:

Rule 16: Never be embarrassed to be full and frank about the details and dimensions of your symptoms, physical and mental. Do not be 'British' about suffering. Do not try to 'Grin and Bear It'. Do not try to 'Keep Calm and Carry On'.

It might sound a small or slight thing, but this turns out to be profoundly important, one of those 'OH, RIGHT!' moments which made me want to write this book, and, hopefully, justifies you reading it. I find myself leaning forward as Juliet's voice softens. She looks tender suddenly, as though her professional distance has fallen away and she is seeing the faces of the thousands of people she has helped and tried to help.

She says, 'It's about when things don't *have* to be alright. So, obviously, we as NHS staff want everybody to feel better. We want people to be better. So that's a *lot* of pressure on you to be better, but maybe you aren't. Maybe it's not alright. And it's *really* important to say so, because it might be the first sign of something going badly wrong. It might be you don't want to disappoint. Even though we want everyone to be better, we want them to be *truly* better and not just saying so. I personally do find that really hard. If I go to a health-care person about a problem, I really struggle if I've gone to them, they've given me an answer and then it hasn't worked; I struggle with going back and saying so. I've regularly not done that. I think that is a British thing: we want to make sure everybody else is happy. But looking after ourselves – it's not going to be mentioned.'

I ask her about different kinds of medication: how does she find the best one?

'Most of the time in mental health, most medications work – they've got the same efficacy but then the side effects are totally different. So say, for example, somebody was a forklift driver, the last thing I want to do is give them medication that makes them sleepy because that messes up their job. If we knew nothing about them except they needed meds and they were a forklift driver, then we would first of all use medication that wasn't sedative. We don't know whether that's going to work for them, but we know that if it does it has a side-effect profile that fits their lifestyle better than anything else.

'Then if you had someone who was highly anxious you would not give them medication that activated them more, so now they were not only anxious, but felt medication was driving them and their anxiety at the same time. If you have very little information about someone, that's how you start to decide about medication – by trying to collect enough information about a person to be able to recommend what might suit them best. It will be about their lifestyle, and what suits that person. So if someone is at a uni, trying to do a degree, then the last thing they want is to be fighting their way through a load of sedation.'

I ask Juliet what information you should give to someone who is prescribing you medication, and what questions you should ask them.

'First of all, you need to know what it is you're looking for. So, your symptoms. And what is it you *want* out of that situation, if you can pull that apart. It's not easy, is it? It might be that your whole life is falling apart and that's as far as you can get. But that's still some information. Then you need to ask what medication choices are there for you, what effects they have, what the differences between them would be, and how much or how little we expect it to make a difference. I think that would be really useful. And setting expectations. I think it is something that we are really bad at. So it would be really powerful if somebody felt able to ask that question. "*What do you expect to change if I take this tablet?*"'

Juliet repeatedly emphasises the value of researching medication, so that you can have an informed conversation with your clinician. If you live in England, she suggests you do it here: choiceandmedication.org/gmmh (this is the Greater Manchester site; your local one will have the initials of your NHS trust after the forward slash).

She says, 'Health-care professionals should know about the problem that you are trying to treat, the possible treatments that work for other people like you, the potential benefits, and risks. And you personally should know about your own values and goals, and they should support you in your preferences. So then if the both of you trust each other and work together, you can come to the decision about medication together, and that's the ideal situation.'

'If you were going to take medication, how would you approach it?' I ask her.

She is unhesitating. 'I would read everything about it. I would use that website. It's written and updated by pharmacists [www.choiceandmedication.org forward slash the initials of your NHS trust]. It tells you things the pharmaceutical companies won't tell you, like whether or not you can drink alcohol with the medication.' (Juliet explains that the corporations err on the side of caution, the general and the worst case, while the pharmacists giving the advice can afford to be more frank, more nuanced and more detailed.)

Juliet adds a note about making sure you are happy with your clinician. 'There are no nurses who are angels, like in the media. And if you find someone that you can work with, that's really good. But you will find people in health care that don't work in a way that you can manage or you can deal with. It would be really nice if you had access to someone when you need it, if you feel you're not being listened to. Like any generalist, you will find GPs who are really good at mental health. The difficulty is, that relies on the GP being the gatekeeper, and *that* relies on the GP knowing when to ask for help.'

This leads us to the regions of labels, language and the limits of medication, beginning with what are still called 'personality disorders' – a label Juliet feels should be binned. 'Personality disorders' include: 'narcissistic' (fragile self-esteem, believing you are special, putting your own needs above others); 'histrionic' (needing to be the centre of attention, being over-dependent on the opinion of others, being easily influenced and feeling you have to entertain, leading to over-dramatic behaviour); 'borderline' (fearing abandonment, experiencing intense and changeable emotion, acting impulsively,

finding it hard to maintain strong and stable relationships); 'avoidant' (avoiding social or work situations
where you will be in the company of others, avoiding
friendships and relationships for fear of rejection, worrying about ridicule, shame, being 'found out', worrying
about attempting activities at which you might embar-
rass yourself); 'dependent' (feeling weak, needy, unable
to function without the support of others, being afraid
of having to rely on yourself and your resources, having
low self-esteem and confidence); 'obsessive-compulsive'
(perfectionism, needing unduly to be in control, fearing
others will make mistakes, setting unrealistically high
standards for yourself and others); and 'personality disorder not otherwise specified' (meaning you do not fit
easily into other 'disorder' categories, but are sufficiently
different – or we could say 'individual' – in some troubling way, leading a clinician to give you this label).
Personally, it only took one reading of this list to convince me that I had every single one of them, either
thinly or deeply buried, or exposed. Don't be alarmed if
this is your experience. The very concepts of personality
and character contain 'disorders'. Thankfully, they contain other things, too.

Juliet says, 'For complex trauma, "complex emotional
needs" is probably the right term – it's a term that doesn't
accuse people of having a disorder or having done
something wrong. There isn't a nice tablet that sorts it
out. Medication probably isn't the answer.

'So suppose we have a person on a huge range of

medication. It isn't going to be sorted by medication, but no one else has anything else to give that person. A lot of my time and energy is spent talking about the fact we have a person who's now on a huge range of medication because they feel mental pain. And it's giving them side effects, but it also validates how they feel. So if we took the medication away, with nothing else instead, we've taken away the only outward sign of their trouble.

'Often the hardest thing is sitting with a person who doesn't really want to stop the medication but isn't benefiting from it. I'm trying to stop that psychological attachment to the medication, and that's a really hard one. And there isn't a lot else out there in the NHS.

'In crisis, if you've got emotions that you cannot manage any longer, then medication can dampen down those emotions, that struggle. Because it *will* make you feel better. But that is part of the [challenge of] managing expectations – I would tell that person they would have that medication but it could only be for three weeks. It's usually three weeks, that's the limit, because it will make you feel better, but after that it's going to be a psychological battle with yourself to come away from that medication. And we hold that line as health-care professionals. And if the person knows that that's coming, then it's still going to be tough, but at least you know it's coming.'

I am amazed by this – so much of what we know and hear about treatment systems involves more medication, not less.

I ask Juliet, 'Is there a reason why people can't just keep taking it for life?'

'So you think it's helping you carry on. Maybe you've developed some coping strategies during that time. Because your emotions have dampened down and you've got some coping strategies. But you think that's the *medication* that's working now – it doesn't, it won't be, it will be your own personal coping strategies. But you don't know that. And you don't value it in yourself, you only value it in the medication, that's the risk. And you value the medication more than yourself. People with complex emotional needs have very low self-esteem, so they're going to find the thing that has made them better, and it may well be they'll name the medication as "the thing". And then of course another crisis comes along. Something happens and it hits you again. And the medication is the thing that has made you better and it obviously isn't working so you need *more* medication. So you go on to more medication, there is nothing else the health service can do, and that helps, it really helps, and then you carry on with your life and now you've found the answer except another crisis *will* come along, because that's life, and that's how people end up on ten medications. Because nobody ever stops the first one. And you, as the person taking the medication, you're thinking, "This is what got me well." But it isn't.'

'What are the best outcomes?' I ask. 'How does someone in serious difficulty best navigate medication?'

Juliet speaks thoughtfully. 'I think it will continue to

dampen your emotions, so that helps, and some people will need to take it long term. Hopefully we will help people early on. If they've got complex emotional needs they'll need to find coping strategies and learn for themselves to manage their emotions, because they didn't pick it up naturally like people with a stable childhood did.'

As we will see, in conversation with a trauma therapist, a great many of us suffer from mental distress as a legacy of early life events. In the model Juliet offers here, medication stabilises the symptoms of this ingrained distress by dampening painful, disturbing or debilitating emotions, and then a therapist helps the sufferer develop daily coping strategies.

Juliet continues, 'If they start early on, and they know there's something that really helps them when they're in a really bad place, and they know that it will help them in the short term, and they stop it again – but in the meantime they learn to use as many skills as they can to make sure that they look after themselves, and learn about the fact that feeling an emotion is not a bad thing, always – then that would be ideal. Then you've always got that first medication to fall back on, and you know that it helps.'

'And so all you need,' I say, emphasising the irony of the 'all', 'is a really good mental health pharmacist and a really good therapist?'

'If we just had as many pharmacists and psychologists as we have nurses and doctors, then I would be happy!'

'And you clearly have a lot of faith in medication,' I say. 'It does work?'

Juliet nods and looks businesslike. 'I've been in mental health since 1994 and I've seen the difference it makes, and I've seen the difference in my family, so yes, it works. And there are times it doesn't need to be used, and maybe we jump too quickly to it. There will be times when medication is definitely *not* the answer, and a lot of the time when we're being asked for advice by GPs we'll be saying, "No, medication is not the answer."

'Often it will be the person: it's not about illness, it's about their life and what's happened to them in their life. So something has just happened, and it's upset them, and they're looking to find a way of not feeling upset. And they're desperate, and the GP goes, "Which medication should I give them to stop feeling upset?"

'And we're saying, "Hmm, actually, feeling upset is a normal way of being. It would be really nice if they could talk to somebody about their problems and think about their coping strategy, but taking a tablet isn't going to resolve any of it." And *awful* things happen to people, really awful, but the medication isn't going to make that any better.'

I ask about care while you are taking the medication. As many people who take – or who have taken – medication know and report, too often you are prescribed a pill and left to get on with it. When should your medication be reviewed?

'What would be really lovely,' Juliet says, 'is if it was

reviewed about six weeks after it was started. You should have a proper review that asks, "Is it helping at all?" And if it isn't, then it shouldn't carry on. And that is what the NICE guidelines say. If you are going to give medication, then you should be reviewing it.

'It's stopping it that's the problem, if it's not working. Actually sitting there and saying, "Right, we've tried this medication, it doesn't work, and I can't think of another that will." That's a real skill: to be able to talk to someone and explain that, actually, those options are not the right options, and what is next. And thinking through what could happen next.'

'And that means therapy and change, doesn't it?' I put in.

Juliet smiles kindly. 'It means hard work. Really hard work, which is really annoying, isn't it? Getting better from a mental health condition can mean really hard work.'

And so, that brings us to . . .

Rule 17: Medication can give you a place to stand: solid mental ground and stabilised emotions. Use that solid ground to make the changes that will make a long-term difference.

It is fortunate that we humans built the pyramids, went to the moon and came up with the plays of Shakespeare, the music of Bach, the *Diary of Anne Frank* and Ada Lovelace's original computer algorithm, or this would start to look like a bit of an ask.

On guesswork and honesty, Juliet says, 'Maybe we're not open enough about guesswork. We should say, "This should work for you," rather than, "This is what you need." And again it comes from desperate want for somebody to get better, rather than some arrogant "I-know-what's-best-for-you". It's more like, "I really want this to make you better so I'm going to tell you so." And then the person takes it. And if they could only feel able to come back and say, "It doesn't really help," or, "It's helped me a bit. Now I can't get out of my chair because I've put on two tons of weight and I'm feeling tired all the time." If there was an easy two-way conversation about medication I think we'd get it right a lot of the time. But there needs to be a whole load of work to get it right.'

It is not just that there are mysteries attached to how medications work, Juliet explains; it is also the case that clinical advice and information can be deliberately bland. There is a reason for this, she says.

'Advice is very generic and very positive, maybe saying, "The tablets are there and they'll help you," because it makes sure that we don't miss the people who are dithering, going, "Actually, I think I can manage without medication . . ." and they struggle on with an awful sad life that might have been transformed by taking a tablet. So if we don't encourage those quiet people who will sit under the radar and never ask for help, then that would be awful. Because it allows people who think medication is the work of the devil, and going to kill them all, to take up all the space – and they're actually very loud.'

She finishes with this thought. 'As soon as staff who work in mental health services start to understand that they are mad too, that would be helpful. I think it is starting to happen. There must be more than one doctor who is ill and has been through tough times recently. We don't hear from them.'

13. Therapy

So, let's suppose you've had the breakdown, or hit the depression, or suffered the anxiety, or fallen into the valley of shadows in any one of the eight billion ways that the 8,000,000,000 humans alive today can fall. You have perhaps sought professional help. You have or have not taken medication. You may be still in the valley of shadows; you may be moving through it; you may be in long-term negotiation with it, or you may be palpably and blessedly over the worst of it. The very fact that you or someone who cares about you is reading this is a good sign: moves are being made. Wherever you have been and wherever you are in the journey through this often dismal place, you or someone close to you is taking action; taking steps towards your recovery and healing. For many of us this involves some form of therapy.

Your path will depend on what is available, how many sessions you can access, what you can afford or afford to queue up for, and whether you find someone who is right for you – or indeed, any good at all.

In various countries – including the UK, France and Nigeria – anyone can call themselves a therapist, advertise and start charging people to talk to them; in most of

Europe and the US you need years of training, and accreditation.

Whether you go for a lot of therapy – a lifetime – a limited course, a few appointments or even a couple of sessions, the experience of therapy is rarely boring. One session with a counsellor at university was extremely helpful: she rapidly identified triggers and advised me how I might avoid and cope with them. When your pride is hurt you need to watch out, she said, when I explained that I had set fire to some bins outside the office of a newspaper which had sacked me. It sounds trite, but I have watched my reactions to hurt pride ever since, and not started any more fires.

Years later, depressed, I turned up to my first session with a therapist, full of suspicion and scepticism, but quite desperate to feel better. When she began asking me about my mother I felt incredulous – my mother? *Really?* Were all the clichés true? They were indeed: she wanted me to talk about my childhood. As it happened, I had written a book about my childhood – wouldn't she rather read that, and save us both a lot of time? She would not. When I was sufficiently disarmed to lower my barriers and commit to telling her the truth and to working with her, we began a shared journey which changed my life infinitely for the better.

In need of therapy, years later, I had an online appointment with one therapist whose reaction to my problems (she told a mutual friend later, stepping over the professional lines therapists aim not to cross) was along the lines of 'Fucking hell!' (Things had become rather complicated; it was OK, I found my way through them, without her.) More recently, I had an appointment with another therapist whose method was to sit and ask occasional questions, and keep reminding us both of the time, which irritated me. She wanted me to tell my story and I felt exhausted and bored at the prospect. I went from her to another who, I felt, was heading towards the comfortable end of a rewarding career, and had heard herself say the things we spoke about too many times before.

So although I have not had any – and I wish I had – for some years, I remain a confirmed fan and advocate of therapy. Interestingly, studies have shown that the modality of therapy you choose – Cognitive Behavioural Therapy, Psychodynamic Therapy, EMDR, et cetera – is less significant than the therapeutic relationship: the chemistry between you and the therapist. You have to be lucky to get the right person, leading you through the right treatment, when you need it. Given the realities of this situation, reading and research, and hearing what therapists themselves have to say, can really help.

Books by therapists and about therapy are an entire industry. I have rarely taught a writing course on which there was not at least one therapist or psychiatrist, looking to turn their experiences into a tome. There are hundreds of thousands of websites, articles and magazines devoted to better well-being, but in the spirit of this guide, I should like to introduce you to an individual who helped me tremendously, who has helped many hundreds of people in trouble – very many of them in the hardest places there are – and who, I am absolutely confident, could help anyone.

She is a remarkable person whose insights and expertise have much to teach. Because we know and trust each other, having worked together, when I asked her to help with this book, my conviction was that if any truly expert therapist was going to be prepared to be bold, frank and fundamental about how we get into trouble and how we might get through it, it would be her. And so it proved.

You may be in therapy already, but in case you are not, or in case you are waiting for a therapist, or in case you cannot find or afford or wait for one, meet this therapist. My aim in our conversations was to unearth the fundamentals: what are the basics that someone in need of therapy might need to know? What do therapists know about healing and recovery, that the rest of us should know?

Our interaction was unusual in that it is rare for a therapist and a former client to meet. Best practice suggests that both need to keep clear boundaries for two to three years after the professional relationship has ended; that a therapeutic relationship is not a friendship; that even after the course of therapy is finished, those boundaries need to be respected and maintained. But when I explained the form and purpose of this guide,

Ellen Sieg PhD, DClinPsych, Principal Clinical Psychologist, currently working in the NHS, agreed to help.

We decided walking and talking would work best. Ellen
is serious about exercise and it was a miserable, cold grey
day at a bleak time of year; the kind of day you really
wish would pass beyond the windows and die in darkness while you curl up under your sofa and whimper – and
therefore exactly the kind of day, if you are serious about
the self-work of recovery, on which you need to go out
and walk.

We meet near the beck, on the edge of the woods
above the town where we both live. I am especially grateful for her trouble now because Ellen has told me she is
having a hard time. She was resolutely positive about her
situation in our exchanges before this encounter, using
phrases like 'making friends with my pain' and 'practising
what I preach'. I am fascinated to know what this might
actually mean, and what her approach might teach.

At first we walk through the bare woods. The sky is
grey, winter rubble grey, the trees slimy wet, and the
undergrowth is tangled wreckage. Ellen is dressed for
hiking, complete with a headband, a small pack and leg
warmers. We talk a little about our lives, about tricky
times, about the winter, cycles and changes. She has just
done a course in Internal Family Systems, a mode of
therapeutic understanding and treatment pioneered by
Richard Schwartz and which fascinates her.

In IFS, the self is understood to be multiple; Ellen
sees this mode of therapy as an adjunct to her work with

Eye Movement Desensitisation and Reprocessing therapy. To explain the way EMDR worked for me when Ellen took me through it: we began with sessions in which we established trust and openness, on my part, and confidence that I was ready to go into traumas I had vaguely outlined, on hers. Then she would either give me two vibrating nodes to hold while I thought about a particularly painful moment or event, or I would tap the arms of my chair and count, or count backwards, or tap and count backwards in French, in order to distract my working memory. At the same time Ellen moved her finger around in the air while I followed it with my gaze, while simultaneously picturing the painful scene or moment.

If you have not come across it before, EMDR probably sounds bonkers. However, the reason why it is funded and recognised by the NHS as an advanced trauma therapy, is because it works. You enter the scene (mine were all forty years old, so old am I) as an observer; you don't exactly feel the same feelings again, but you are aware of them. And you pick up more feelings and atmospheres around that moment, as though your powers of recall have suddenly become supercharged, and you seem to see it again, more deeply and more fully, more brightly and (much) more calmly than the ways in which you experienced it at the time. It is as though you are an adult watching the distressed child of yourself, not unmoved, of course (I burst into tears aplenty, and each time I cried a *lot*), but able to see the scene for what it was – a child in a miserable and frightening position – rather than how you experienced it, as a downpour of shame, insecurity and fear.

Ellen's way of measuring the success of each session was to ask me how and where I felt a reaction in my body before and after we set about a memory sequence. It felt like unearthing dirty crystals, my buried pains and insecurities, and smashing them, and 'dirty crystals' became our shorthand. So when we first addressed one – a scene of tension and argument in the car on the motorway, when I was six, say – the memory would give me a knot of tension in the pit of my stomach, and I would rate it at eight out of ten for strength. By the end of multiple sessions (we would address the same memory repeatedly) the ratings were all down to two or three; my stomach would feel physically different, largely unbothered, when I thought about the scene. I would recommend anyone to seek EMDR treatment – it is available for trauma on the NHS. If you have been given any one of various 'personality disorder' diagnoses (for an outline of this class of diagnosis, see pages 178–9), you could point out to your GP that these are being reframed as 'complex emotional needs', linked to trauma, and ask for a referral.

Ellen is now pursuing Internal Family Systems. In IFS, childhood trauma can lead to 'exiled emotions': pain, fear, sadness and anger can become 'exiles'.

We deal with them through 'managers', parts of the mind and behaviour which influence the ways we react to and interact with the world; managers are seeking to protect and shield us from being overwhelmed by the pain and trauma of exile.

The third part of the mind, in this model, is composed of 'firefighters', which are reactive thoughts and behaviours, triggered when the pain and demands of our exiles threaten to break out or dominate. So drink, drugs, overwork, compulsive or impulsive behaviours can all be understood as firefighters.

Ellen clearly finds the model useful. There are many different kinds of therapy, including cognitive, psychodynamic, existential, interpersonal; and every therapist develops and tweaks their own version of the kind they offer. She is a specialist trauma therapist who uses EMDR in her work for the NHS, and in private practice. She explains that the aim of IFS is to help people have greater access to 'self-energy' by befriending the exiles, understanding and appreciating the firefighters, and working towards an internal system that appreciates and accommodates the multiplicity of the self, which, in an easy mind, leads and directs us.

Achieving a system that works relatively harmoniously with its multiple parts, she says, can require long-term therapeutic work, especially when exiles are loaded with traumatic memories from a troubled childhood.

We arrive at the National Trust café in the woods, get tea and chocolate – one of her firefighters, Ellen says – and when we are settled at a table outside, I open my notebook.

'What are the fundamentals of trauma and healing,' I ask, 'as a therapist like you understands them?'

'The concept of self,' she says, immediately. 'If you've got enough sense of self, you can almost treat yourself. Most people have attachment-related issues – I do, you do – it goes back to our parents and carers. And stability. Stability is great! Changes to stability are where the problems lie.' Then she observes, 'In private therapy you treat a lot of functioning people; it is when people are *not* functioning that you see them in the health-care system.'

Her inference here is that in order to find, book, pay for and turn up to a private appointment you need to be capable of a tricky, exacting and expensive operation. But if you are broke and in bits you are more likely to come to therapy because someone else arranges and funds it – the NHS.

'But in both cases so much of it comes down to ACEs – adverse childhood experiences. If you have adverse childhood experiences you are far more likely to have adverse mental health. ACEs can be physical or sexual abuse, poverty, a bad experience of moving house, poor friendships, a bad neighbourhood – friendships and neighbourhoods make a huge difference. We do not all start out the same. Some money behind you really does help. And so does your parents'/caregivers' capacity to see and emotionally nourish you.

'And then there is neglect. We talk about sexual abuse as if it's not comparable to anything, but you can't compare pain. If you haven't been *seen* as a child, if you haven't been fully appreciated and seen, reflected, seen and loved – if that's not there, that's neglect.'

This makes sense to me: a neglected child, who was not really heard, seen, loved, listened to, validated, played with. A child who has not been fully and supportively loved, can become a damaged and desperate adult. Sexual abuse enacts the same violence on the mind and soul.

'Your sense of self is constantly evolving. If your parents don't look at you, then shame starts to happen. And it can go very deep into the sense of self. It's not fair, but some people need to work much harder to establish and maintain good levels of mental health.'

Developing her previous point, Ellen is talking here about levels of resilience laid down in early childhood. A stable, loving and supported upbringing in which you are not shamed, confused, made to feel guilty, unimportant, unloved or uncared for, gives a bedrock of strength, a sense of yourself and a sense of self-reliance.

'If women are raped in war, if they have a good sense of self, if they have good attachment behind them from when they were growing up, they have a much better chance of recovery. They don't sublimate the evil into themselves and blame themselves for it. And if we have attachment-related issues we can overcompensate, which becomes narcissism.

'And of course we are all brilliant! But it's much lovelier if we know that early on. In natural disasters people who have good networks recover from pain and loss.

What is difficult are the childhood wounds which cloud over your identity.

'In Internal Family Systems, identity is the sun and the cloudy parts are your exiled feelings, the "I'm not good enough". The aim of the therapy is that you can get back in the sun, that the self isn't damaged, just clouded over.'

She pauses.

Then she says, 'In therapy we hold out a hand. We try to help you to say, "This is me, I'm hurting, and that's not bad, that doesn't make me bad – it's OK, it's right."

'So the aim is that the sense of self and safety feels *bigger* than me. Because my sense of self is in *connection* – it's not separate. I'm not separate – so if I am a child, I can rely on Mum and Dad. Even when I'm bad, they *see* me. It fits with Buddhism – there's something bigger than you in which you are held. IFS fits with many religious ideas – that there is something bigger than us that we can have direct access to.

'Emotions become exiled, for example, if when you are a child it's never safe to feel really sad. What does a child do if they're not allowed to cry or feel anxious? In the way IFS understands it, you develop managers – if you feel part of you is not seen or helped or loved, you shut it up – you repress all this doubt and shame about yourself. And so a good therapist brings that out. That part of you *is* lovable and I show that to you. You need to appreciate that hurt child inside you and love him as much as your own child,' she says, and I know she is talking to me as much as she is to you, dear reader.

If you have been in a place of self-loathing, or of loathing what your life seems to have become, and if you have turned the hate and pain of those feelings upon yourself, blaming yourself for your choices, your situation, your pain, then Ellen is telling you – a whole world of therapy is telling you – that we all carry our child selves inside us, and that shutting down that child's pain, or blocking it out, or blaming yourself for the feelings it produces, are not the right responses. That child needs love, needs help, needs hearing and caring – and that is what a great therapist is for. This is so fundamental to the understanding and treatment of so much of our suffering that it is worth stating again, and absorbing, and remembering:

> **Rule 18: We all carry our child selves inside us. Shutting down that child's pain, or blocking it out, or blaming yourself for the feelings it produces, are not the right responses. That child needs love, help, hearing and care. That child needs therapy.**

'Can you explain what you mean,' I say, 'by "making friends with your pain"?'

'People block emotions,' Ellen says. 'They might be in touch with their emotions but they're scared of them. We block emotions because we think we can't handle them. But if you don't block them, something so beautiful can happen. Emotion is like a great wave of energy, and you can extend your window of tolerance to it. You can enjoy it and notice it. Learn to look after that part of yourself. Don't fight it. Befriend it. Bring it back. And when I'm down I tell myself that is what I have to do: if I can get in touch with that sadness and love it. If you have trauma from your childhood it's often that you had no one to negotiate your emotions with you, so you have to do it as an adult.'

She grins wryly at me. 'This is why I gave you diaries to note down how you were feeling. I knew you wouldn't do it! But what they're for is to help you notice what you're doing. So, for me, I might say to myself, "Jesus, you ran all this distance, you went dancing – calm down!" It's about taking yourself extremely seriously and notic-ing what you are doing and what you are feeling.'

When I first went to see Ellen as a client I was extremely adept at repressing aspects of myself and my life which were harming me and those around me, blam-ing myself for my pain and trouble, and cracking on. Or rather, I was extremely *practised* at it. In the end, this method led me to the mental hospital. Practising what she preaches is professionally and personally invaluable to Ellen – she is in the habit of watching her own behav-iours, habits and choices dispassionately, interrogating them ('Why am I running so much?' 'What is driving all this running and dancing?' 'What do I really want?' 'What do I need – now, tomorrow, next week, in my wider life?') and making changes. She constantly urged me to listen to myself, especially in stressful situations, to ask what I needed, and to make adjustments. So, for example, she urged me to tell my family when I was stressed, when I needed space, when I needed to do less or more or different. I now apply these questions and changes to my work and life as much as I can. It often means saying, 'No (thank you / sorry).' It has taken me decades to say 'no' and not feel guilty.

In my case, Ellen points out, when I need looking after, my first response is to go off and look after someone else. While she was working with me, Ellen was particularly vigilant and forceful about shame. Now she says, 'I hate shame. Shame is really *shit*. And shame is complicated – a secondary emotion – you judge yourself for having needs or emotions.'

In other words – I feel angry, because someone has wronged me. A primary emotion. And then I feel ashamed of myself for feeling angry – a secondary emotion. But what so riles the therapist in Ellen is that the primary emotion is where the truth is, where the need is: in that anger there is validity, meaning and the potential for hope through help and change. If you then subsume that primary anger into shame, you double the problem – the emotion becomes 'exiled'.

'Dance and somatic body movement practices can be really helpful to recognise and befriend exiled emotions, so you can integrate them, or at least learn to appreciate them, without replicating the unhelpful judgements that we have been shamed with in our childhood.

'We're so phobic of emotion. This is why I dance so

much. When I dance, it takes me to a place where I am calm and dreamy. It's about allowing yourself to feel without judging yourself for those feelings. We need to make room for the exiles, the emotions, the feelings. Because when you have those exiled emotions, that's when you might do something else to not feel them.'

As is clear, Ellen places huge emphasis on the relationship between the body and the mind. Doing EMDR with her was a mindfully physical experience. 'Where in your body do you feel that?' she would ask, as we addressed a painful or difficult or shame-making memory. 'How does it feel to think about it, on a scale of one to ten?'

'What is so important about EMDR,' she says now, 'is because it is a bridge between the body and the mind. We hold emotion in the body. We need to befriend that physically. Where is it? What does it have to teach us – where do you feel it in the body? CBT is useful but it's so cognitive, it's all here,' she says, gesturing, 'in the head.'

Cognitive Behavioural Therapy focuses on mental strategies, retraining your thought patterns. Although CBT therapists advocate exercise and physical activity, of course, CBT is much more a mental than a physical therapy.

I press Ellen about that phrase she used, 'making friends with my pain', since it seems such a potentially powerful idea. As she talks I begin to see she is using the idea of friendship in a particular way; it is as though she is recruiting her pain to help her, to push her forward, forging an alliance with it, rather than allowing it to crush or limit her.

'The way I do it is through dance, noticing, nature, being in my body. If I'm in touch with a lot of emotion it's very helpful to allow myself to feel it rather than blocking it. Go *into* it – once you feel secure enough to hold it.'

Considering how this approach might apply to individual forms of suffering, I thought of the death of my sister. The grief would come out of nowhere in dreadful, debilitating waves. There was no way of denying, avoiding or suppressing it: I could only howl on the inside and cry on the outside. I had no choice but to sit with it, as it were – to go through it, to feel it intensely and utterly until it subsided.

The great Israeli writer David Grossman said that in the storm of misery he felt at the death of his son, 'I thought, "this is a human experience and I am going to experience it".'

This is my best understanding of 'befriending' your pain. With anxiety, for example, sufferers report that rather than trying to fight it, to flee it, to fear it, a more successful approach is to embrace it. To follow its fears to their ultimate, absurd conclusion ('What is the very worst that could happen?'); to be open about it, to actively tell people about it (as I do with my seasonal depressions), to see it not as a monster that cannot be killed but as an idiosyncratic side of a multiple and colourful self, part of the constellation of qualities and quirks which are the unique being that is you, something which sits beside all the blessings and beauties which people love and admire and even envy in you.

Befriending the pain of depression, for me, means not hiding from it, not denying it, and not being crushed by it. Rather, it means seeing my depression as something which also makes me more sensitive, more understanding, more honest, more brave, and more determined, when depressed, to do the things which I know are soothing to it, and good for me, even and especially when all I want to do is lose myself in the internet, box sets or movie streaming sites indefinitely, until it somehow buggers off.

It sounds absurdly trite to say to someone suffering from an eating disorder, for example, that they should 'make friends with their pain'. But two highly successful and inspirational people I know, both expert and admired mental health professionals, who have both lived through life-threatening bouts of anorexia, both now talk about those times and the ways in which they manage their lives now, the pressures they work with and the pulses of fear that their disorder might return, exactly as though they have indeed taken the painful distress which drove them to starve themselves and folded it into the embrace of how they see themselves and who they are. When they talk about being treated in the psychiatric system and the changes they have made and the strategies they follow, the ways in which they monitor and take care of themselves, it is not at all as though they are talking about a disease or a loss or a damage. It is more like listening to someone describing a careful approach to a delicate relationship – a relationship which means a lot to them, which is important to their lives, but which does not define them.

'Go into it once you feel secure enough to hold it,' I put in. 'Once you feel secure enough? That's a lot.'

'That's why you need a good therapist,' Ellen responds, 'if you have not got enough self to do that work. So it's about uncovering the clouds and moving them off the sun. EMDR and IFS are based on the principle that if I create the right conditions you will heal yourself. The good news about therapy and self-help is you can get back to the sun. You can get back to yourself and access your energy. I create the environment so that you feel loving enough, protected enough. I extend my hand to you and then we can go through it together.'

'How do you go about building up the self, for yourself?' I ask.

'For me?' she says. 'I do breath work. Meditation.'

Breath work is the practice of consciously controlling your breathing in order to alter – to calm – your mental state. One of my friends, a successful actor who went through breakdown long ago, is in the habit of using a long, slow out-breath, like a protracted and silent whistle, to ease and tranquillise her feelings in the moment, in everyday stressful situations. I have adopted the same trick and find it very useful. When I began acting as a child, my mother – who was (is, privately) an accomplished actress – told me to take three deep breaths just before going onstage. 'Cool, calm and collected,' she advised – effectively a meditative mantra. It seemed to work, though now it is generally believed that breathing out slowly is more calming than breathing in.

'You can't take the protectors away before you have something else to replace them with,' Ellen explains. 'Let's say, for you, your protector is a bottle of wine. So it's your firefighter: you feel the emotions and you reach for wine, or chocolate. If I take that away, what do you do then, with that emotion? So we do stabilising work. We bring in Wise Figures and Protectors. A Wise Figure could be the Dalai Lama, it could be a friend. And we bring in Protectors – protectors could be a friend, an imaginary being, a persona, like a lion, an inner protector. And we need Nurturers – a nurturer could be a fairy godmother, a made-up figure, a friend. So you come to think, I have helpers. I have a nurturer, and she's going to sort me out. She will sit with me when I'm depressed. If I am in trouble I can draw on them, or I can make them up, bring them in and draw on them.'

Ellen continues, 'Women who have been abused need a lot of protectors. We do breath work, for anxiety. For depression it is so important. And it is really important you do the things that make you feel good when you are fine, when you're *not* feeling good. So they become less of a first-aid kit and more of a way of life.'

These protectors and wise figures might sound rather

abstract, or somewhat airy-fairy, if only because I am asking Ellen to summarise the process and these various imagined characters, rather than going through the work and creating them.

But as she speaks, I think of my mother and father, nurturing individuals I have been hugely fortunate to be able to draw on – as themselves and at a distance, as figures, in fact and in thought – throughout my life.

I think of my father, a wise figure if ever there was one, who was always and is still a protecting, counselling, guiding presence, even though he was absent for much of my childhood, whose influence and nurturing have in no way diminished since he died in 2019.

And I think of my sort-of-stepfather, Gerard Morgan-Grenville, the love of my mother's life, whom she met years after she and my father separated, who became a friend, a mentor, a kind of godfather to me.

When in difficulty, in doubt or in happiness, I think often of him and of my father, of what they would say, of how they would throw lightness and humour along with seriousness and concentration at a problem, of their faith in themselves and their faith in me.

With them in mind, what Ellen is saying could not be less airy-fairy. They were both extremely shrewd, clever, daring and funny men. All the lessons, ideas and ways of thinking they taught me, either explicitly or by example, have been mighty powers and advantages to me, always. I cannot report, stage by stage, how a course of therapy in IFS might feel and change things, but I feel I can absolutely appreciate how it works.

The link between the body and mind, and the emphasis Ellen places on the physical as a route to our thoughts and feelings, is powerful when you work with her, and intriguing. What is the role of the body, of physical interventions, like Prince Harry's famous arms-crossed shoulder-tapping (an exercise Ellen had me do)?

'If someone is highly anxious, then their nervous system is overstimulated – it needs to calm down. Music can be really helpful, and breath work. Calm music. And if you are down, if you are in some kind of withdrawal, then of course music – life – energy! Tapping is helpful for processing. It distracts the working memory. It's really calming.'

Now I ask Ellen about looking after herself while she treats people. How does one balance the two? The key, she explains, is the difference between empathy and compassion.

'You give more if you give yourself more,' she says. 'If I am using empathy when I am working with some-one who has had terrible experiences, if I am "feeling for" them, it can be too much. You burn out. But if I am using compassion, feeling *with* them, then I can do it; I can help and protect myself at the same time. So if I'm working with someone and she is blocking her emo-tions, if I'm using empathy I feel it. I feel that blocking inside me, too. But if I am being compassionate, then I would be feeling *with* her. So we use helpful listening. Helpful listening is about presence. People are starved of presence, especially people in distress. So you really tune in to them. You give them your full presence, giving them all your attention. And if I can tune in to what you are feeling, what you are saying, you feel *seen*. What is important is not your story, but that I'm with you. You're seen. I strongly tune in to you, which means I am fully present and listening.'

Ellen's point is that compassion allows the listener, the helper, to maintain what Ellen calls 'self-energy', which very high levels of empathy – 'suffering for' – would deplete, harming the listener and the help they are able to give.

'The more self-energy you have,' Ellen says, 'the more you can do. If I am strong, then I'm much more present; I have more self available. A really good therapist can feel how you are as you come into the room, and they tap in to how that person is. If I find they are very depressed, I see them, I offer space, I make space for them to talk, but I don't do too much. It's a relationship. You remind them you're there, you listen, you really listen, but you don't feel you have to fix them.'

Mike Slade, a world-leading recovery expert (whom we encountered in Chapter 11 and will meet in the next chapter), and John Mitchell, a specialist in talking to people in the most dire difficulty, make the same point:

the feeling of having to fix someone, especially someone to whom you are very close, is painfully hard to bear and agonising to attempt to enact. But however much we might feel driven to do it, or to attempt it, people who study it professionally insist it is not our role: it is not even clear that it is possible. However, we can – we must and we can – find ways to help people fix themselves.

One of the ways in which psychiatry has gone wrong, it seems to me, is the expectation of 'fixing' people which our system places on psychiatrists and medication. Clearly this is to the enormous advantage of the profession and the pharmaceutical corporations, in terms of cash, power and prestige, but no psychiatrist is likely to claim that they can 'heal' you: treat you and improve your quality of life, reduce your symptoms, yes – but hopes of 'fixing' or 'healing' are more ideas that we sufferers bring to our clinicians than they are claims that individual psychiatrists would privately make. At the same time, they would not want to disabuse you of any belief in your recovery that you might have – because those beliefs are vital. Although psychiatry and medication can be wonderfully effective in alleviating symptoms and suffering, they are rarely if ever able to heal anyone – and the language, framing and expectations our model sets for sufferers, that there is something 'wrong' that can be made 'right' along with side effects and stigma, can and does actively harm recovery.

So if you are suffering, or you have suffered, rather

than longing and pining for an imagined future in which you no longer have any symptoms – as in resetting and stabilising a broken bone, and looking forward to it healing – you might well find that deciding to live with and through your condition, making changes around it and aiming to grow through and with those changes, is a more successful strategy. As we will see in the following chapters, everything we know and can measure about recovery supports this. Embrace, however horrible the feelings are, rather than deny. Because frankly admitting to yourself that your troubles are part of you is the first stage of coping with them, and leads to the second: action.

Suddenly Ellen grins and mimes throwing a ball at me – something she did once, in a session. The idea is to jerk you out of your inner confinement, playfully, and return you to the present, to the moment, to reality.

'Or I'll throw a ball!' she says. 'You're back! Ah, *there* you are! Don't *judge*.'

(She used to say this to me in our sessions, implicitly and explicitly, when I was down and beating myself up inside.)

'We've been trained to feel so much shame. We shame ourselves for strong emotions. Why should we do this, rather than celebrate people's capacity to feel! We should think, "OK, I'm a person who can feel a lot." It doesn't make you a bad person. It makes you a very colourful person.'

There are reams, entire libraries more to be said and

read about therapy. But such are some of the basics, anyway, from the best therapist I can imagine.

Rule 19: You are going to do most of your own healing, and for that you need a strong sense of self. There are ways of building up that sense (this book is full of them). Get to it.

14. The self-work of recovery

You could scarcely ask for a more glum and greasy morning than the one on which she appeared, though there had been plenty of competition recently. The winter brings days smothered in trawler nets of rain, days which seem crushed in the fist of the darkest time of the year. The only hopeful glimpses of blue sky come in small spills of unexpected light, leaking out of the grip of dull noons and wet, dim dusks. The jackdaws were making disbelieving remarks on the approach of another dripping squall (they have a tremendous, unflagging sense of humour) when a figure came down the road. She was retired, I would guess; white-haired, stepping carefully and quickly; she was dressed in efficient waterproofs. In her left hand she carried a white sack and in her right a litter picker. She worked quickly, the picker dipping and gripping and depositing with a deft, busy motion, like a sparrow raiding a bird table. No one had asked her to do it, and no one was paying her to do it, but she had decided to clear rubbish, the tattered scraps and the refuse of recycling, out of the gutters and off the pavements of wherever her walk through town would take her. Across northern Europe it is thought that at least 12 million people suffer from winter blues, but that figure is drawn from those who report it. The actual proportion of the population who feel our hopes and spirits dip with the dark is unknown – what do you guess: half? Three-quarters?

(I have only met one man who said the winter was his favourite season, and that was on a thrilling, frozen night in the deep cold; we were in a warm pub for a poetry reading and he was duffled up in the perfect coat and scarf.)

Adding this season to any kind of trouble in the mind or body makes the landscape, inner and outer, start to sprout despair. You see it in the angle of people's heads, downward-looking, as if scanning for puddles.

What was so striking about the litter picker was her posture. A dozen people had been up and down the road that morning, all in rain gear, some in hats, most in hoods, one holding a shawl over her head. The lines of their bodies and the way they held themselves were all hunched, head down in resistance. My neighbour walked defiantly, his hood streaming, his face scrunched up. There was rejection and resentment in every figure – you could read the thought bubbles over their heads, *Bloody, bloody rain.* And you knew the rain was standing in for a world of worry – pressure, prices, work, health, cuts, strikes, flu, the war. It was a right miserable time to be alive, or so it seemed then.

But not to the litter picker! The wet weight of a morning that oppressed the rest of the town – the spatter of guttering, the slop-splash of passing cars, the clammy scrabbling of drab, remorseless wet and grey cold – was the very thing that seemed to power her. She moved straight-backed, with concentration. You would have to say it – she looked mindful, and mindfully alive. She was not experiencing the vile conditions as a trial, as yet another thing to overcome, as yet another reason not to be especially happy, or not to be happy at all. On the contrary, she was alert, and busy, challenging and changing the world, and the fact that the elements and the very soul-weather of the day were gruelling and tiresome underlined what she was doing, made it all the better, made it all the stronger, made it an even greater service to the town and to herself than if it had been sunny and all the birds a-singing. The litter picker is a perfect example of turning something oppressive into something uplifting, and this is what this chapter is about.

The good news is, we now know a huge amount about recovery, how it works and how to go about it. There is no bad news, except that it requires work – and this is some of the most interesting and rewarding work you will ever do, and the rewards are far greater than money (though money may well be a side benefit).

A world authority on the subject is Mike Slade, Professor of Mental Health Recovery and Social Inclusion at the University of Nottingham. Mike works at the sharp end of the spectrum in that he targets his research specifically at psychosis and, especially, schizophrenia. The reason for this, he told me, is that psychiatry and the mental health systems take these serious conditions extremely seriously: progress there ripples out rapidly and becomes progress in the much more common areas of depression, anxiety, OCD, eating disorders and so-called 'personality disorders' (as I have said already, a hateful phrase which sensitive professionals are abandoning in favour of 'complex emotional needs').

If you want to refocus the entire system, which Mike does, then addressing it at the crucial points of schizophrenia and psychosis is the way to drive wholesale and widespread systemic change, he believes. So regardless of whether you have experienced schizophrenia or psychosis, or whatever you are suffering or have suffered from, the tools and approaches Mike has trialled and developed are also very much for you. Anyone who has suffered distress or difficulty, be it mild, moderate or severe, should know about the CHIME framework, developed by Mike and his teams. CHIME stands for:

- Connectedness
- Hope
- Identity
- Meaning
- Empowerment.

It is now the most widely used system, internationally, to understand and operationalise what recovery means.

For someone at the start of a recovery journey – and you can start this as soon as you feel low – you might think about beginning by rejecting a lot of what the internet, the prevailing culture and the health system might make you feel by telling you what you should feel.

Or, as Mike puts it, 'A system that tells me how everything is hopeless, and I should abandon my life ambitions, and accept my identity as a "mental health service user", and live with the stigma and discrimination that entails, and recognise that it's useful to be disconnected from other people so you can recover and then get back into life later – and all other toxic kinds of assumptions – are challenged by people with experiential knowledge.'

Mike naturally speaks like the former clinician, lecturer, academic, researcher and international authority that he is. Decoded, 'challenged by people with experiential knowledge' can be read to mean: 'The story you are being told about the implications of mental suffering and what it might mean for your life, and the actual lives of sufferers, are two different things. And the doom narrative is bullshit.'

From the forefront of recovery research comes this simple message:

Rule 20: What happens to you is not about anyone else's narrative. It's about yours. Do not tell yourself a story which dooms you to suffering. Do the work you need to live and tell a story of recovery.

Mike's work blossoms with ambition and momentum – with a team of thirty-seven researchers from Nottingham University and King's College London he is currently bidding for an enormous grant to start a centre, based

on 'disruptive innovation' according to the funding criteria, which aims to switch around the thinking on
mental health from how we should treat illness to how
we should promote strong well-being, increase protective factors, support resilience and build mentally healthy
communities and societies.

What is a healthy community? My favourite example
of what might otherwise seem a nebulous concept is the
French city of Grenoble. From the Socialists and the
Greens, who fought each other at the polls but who
shared similar policies and visions, came a list of ideas
for the future of the city which citizens were invited to
vote upon. The first winner was a proposal to remove all
advertising from the city. And so they did. If you own a
shop you can still advertise in the window, to about A4
size. Otherwise, the only adverts are public information
notices. And so the trams, the walls, the windows, those
green pillars on the pavements that the French like, normally covered in ads, the bus stops and tram stops – none
of it tries subtly to undermine you in order to sell you
something. And here is the strange thing: when you
arrive in Grenoble, before you know what the difference
is, the city feels wonderfully calm and easy. There is a
kind of peace in the air which is hard to understand or
pin down until you realise – no ads! And then there is
the genius of the scheme: the argument for doing away
with the whole slurry of advertising, throughout the
whole city, was made on the grounds of children's mental
health. From the start, now, the children of Grenoble

are brought up in a city whose surfaces do not lie to them, undermine them or try to hard-sell them anything. This is the kind of change Mike plans to investigate: *how might we do it all differently?*

The most striking thing about Mike's work is that you do not know about it already: the mental health systems of different countries are advancing at different speeds towards very different places – as we will see, Belgium and Finland are much further ahead than Britain, for example. Your children and grandchildren will understand mental health very differently from the way we do now, and that will be partly thanks to people like Mike Slade and the work they are currently doing, and partly, one would hope, down to countries which are lagging behind adopting the approaches of more progressive ones.

The success and the speed with which the ideas and contentions of Nottingham's Institute of Mental Health are being proven and adopted would seem to prove Mike's fundamental conviction correct: listen to the people who have been there, redesign the system using what they have found and what they tell you, concentrate on what makes people well, and recovery, rather than on simply managing (or not) illness, and the whole thing will work better.

It is worth understanding how this change is taking place. Mike explains that who we listen to depends on how we value what they have to say, which in turn depends on the language they use, and whether our academic and clinical systems regard that language as objective, scientific and evidence-based.

'Different types of value are placed on different types of knowers,' he says. 'So if I'm a clinician working with someone with depression I do an "objective assessment". In other words, I look at the person and write down what I see – that's an "objective" assessment. If I'm listening to what the person themselves says, and writing *that* down, that's a "subjective" assessment. So the subjective is, "The person said, 'I feel miserable.'" The objective is, "They had slow behaviour and spoke in a low and emotional way." The very *language* devalues experiential knowledge and privileges the knowledge of the – in quotes – "expert". So in some ways [our work here] is the translation of experience into a legitimate form of knowledge.'

The CHIME framework is being adopted internationally, precisely because Mike and his teams have been able to translate what sufferers have been telling them into evidence-based clinical knowledge that systems and institutions are able to accept.

I asked Mike to take me through the elements of CHIME.

First, **connectedness**. In Finland, he told me, as a response to lockdown and the isolation brought about by the pandemic, a group started a CHIME choir.

'They're collective, they're experiential, so they're about doing, not thinking, they're bringing people together, they're amplifying their strengths and goals: they do all these recovery-related things. And of course it has an attraction for people with lived experience of mental health-related issues, but it's not solely for them.'

Mike points out that a member of a CHIME choir is not thinking of themselves as someone with a mental health problem – they're thinking of themselves as part of a choir, a tribe, a group. Connectedness is key here, and perhaps more subtle and various than it might appear, and perhaps less off-putting than it might seem if, like me, you are naturally shy. Connectedness can grow from the obvious places – joining a group of people with similar interests, attending events – or it can begin in more sidelong ways. The litter picker may not have spoken with anyone, that morbid morning, but on a fairer day she surely would have done, had she wished to, and in any case her altruism was forming a connection with her community and her place within it which, research has shown, really works.

A small study by the University of Ohio took 122 people suffering moderate or severe depression, anxiety or stress and measured how they felt after taking part in one of three activities.

One group was given a Cognitive Behavioural Therapy technique, keeping diaries of their thoughts in order to recognise and change negative patterns. The second group was asked to do social activities, planning and taking part in two per week, with other people, 'for the purposes of enjoyment', and the third group was asked to perform three random acts of kindness to others, twice a week. The acts were defined as big or small, costing a small amount of time or resources.

The results showed a large and marked impact on the random kindness group, a smaller but marked effect on the CBT group, and a similar though smaller effect on the socialisers. This story was published in the *Journal of Positive Psychology* and picked up by a newspaper, and then disappeared, as these things do.

But the implications are enormous. Before we think about self-work as a looking inwards, a concentration on strategies to make the body and mind happier, consider this:

Suppose a fundamental part of the self is the other: not just those others known to us and who mean so much to us, but the wide, wide world of unknown friends.

In China, altruism is a subject of scholarly research. The feeling among Chinese scholars is that the link between altruism and well-being is known in individualistic Western societies, but not established in China's collectivist society, as it transitions to a form of hypercapitalism. If you have seen ambulances blocked in the mega-traffic of a Chinese city, traffic which is too concerned with its own problems to get out of the way, you will appreciate their point. Studies carried out there yield astonishing results.

One asked an unexpected question: does helping other people make you feel *warmer*? Physically warmer. Researchers looked at people who helped others during

the Hurricane Sandy disaster in the US, and then repli-
cated crisis situations in a lab. As the researchers
commented, 'While improving the welfare of others,
altruistic behaviours typically deplete the energy and
resources of the altruistic performers.' But then they
did the experiments, rigorously, and, 'We found an
immediate rewarding effect on the perceived warmth of
the ambient environment after performing altruistic
behaviours.'

The extraordinary fact is, performing an act of kindness, doing something for someone else, actually changes
the world you inhabit, or at least your experience of it,
which might as well be the same thing.

A second study confirmed the first: altruism was
found to directly and indirectly promote well-being. The
indirect element comes about because doing a good turn
to someone else changes the way you feel about yourself. 'People who help others reap elevated self-esteem,
which in turn serves as a proximate mechanism that
facilitates well-being,' the researchers concluded. Perhaps we have always known this, innately, but it is rather
wonderful that it has been proved.

Rule 21: To help yourself, help others.

No wonder the litter picker looked more chipper,
more alert and happier than everyone else who walked
down the road that morning. She was warmer, for a
start.

*

The second element of CHIME is **hope**, which turns out to be one of the most powerful forces in recovery. When I ask Professor Mike Slade to talk to me about hope, he begins with a story about a failed funding bid. (It's a lot more fun than it sounds.)

'The concept of hope and diagnostic frameworks are not very compatible,' he says. 'We put in a bid a while ago and one of the criteria we were proposing to measure was the degree of hope experienced by research subjects. The panel turned us down with a phrase I will never forget: "Hope is not a sufficiently important clinical outcome!" The idea that hope is a passing feeling, not a clinical outcome!'

Mike becomes delightfully animated, even by the standards of a naturally animated man, passionate about his work and communicating his discoveries. Had we been sitting at a table, he would have banged his hand on it.

'Every one of us knows that recovery begins when you find a glimmer of hope!'

'How do we make it, then?' I ask. 'Where does hope come from?'

'What supports hope?' he returns. 'Role models. That's why peer support work is so vital in recovery. We *know* the conversations we have, the language we use, supports or reduces hope. So when we encourage the lowering of expectations, or in psychiatric parlance, "realistic expectations" – they're *always* lower, they're never higher – what we're actually doing is *reducing hope*. We're damaging the person.

'Suppose someone has "unrealistic aspirations" – so, something that from my perspective as a clinician is very unlikely to happen – well, my view *doesn't matter*. It's their life. So as a clinical psychologist in the Maudsley I had a patient with psychosis. And I was working with a guy and it became clear his main goal in life was to become an MP. The standard approach would be to lower expectations.

'So I said, "OK, what are the stepping stones to getting there?" There is an immediate power shift if you do that – now he has something to contribute. So we worked through it. How is he going to raise the money to get on the ballot paper? How is he going to deal with hecklers? What is his manifesto? And he got on to the ballot! And he stood in the general election. I had to decide whether to vote for him.

'*This* is what recovery support is about. It is not about *fixing* the person or making them "normal". Because that's not a goal put on any other citizen, is it? Entrenched in that idea of fixing someone or making them normal is a discriminatory, stigmatised view.

'Everyone *else* needs to follow their dreams, amplify their strengths, live in a supportive community, have friends, have lovers, have jobs – but *this* group, this group needs treatment, and then they'll be ready for all this other stuff. I think it's the fundamental mistake with this model. People live up to or down to the expectations that are put on them.'

We began this guide with the idea that language frames your understanding of your position, of what has happened to you, and therefore your expectations of what will or might happen to you, of what can or should happen to you. And of course those expectations are hugely powerful – not just in determining your fate, but in setting the range and possibilities of your fate.

Talking to Mike reinforces the sense that the interlocked struts of language, hope and outcome are fundamental parts of better well-being, a keel of the whole ship of healing. He describes how people are exploring reframing their experiences in order to overcome them, and the ways in which our current system reacts or resists.

'We have a PhD student currently submitting her thesis on what psychiatry would label as a "mental health-related breakdown", and on relabelling that as "spiritual emergence". And so she is looking at what happens when people provide that – a spiritual emergence – as an entirely alternative frame of reference. We've done some really interesting work on the struggles that people have to frame what society gives them as mental health issues, but what they experience, as individuals, as spiritual issues.'

Imagine you are suffering acute depression, or vicious, overwhelming anxiety, or suppose you are experiencing such intense misery and mental pain that only self-harm seems to alleviate it. You don't want to see anyone and you can't possibly go to work: you can barely get out of the bedroom, never mind the house. Through a wonderfully incisive intervention by someone who cares about you, or a mighty, mighty effort of your own, you make it to the doctor. And the doctor asks you what is happening in your life. She enquires after your home and family situation, your work or your studies. She asks, delicately, if there is something particular that might be causing you pain. As Dr Kate Kerr did, she makes judgements – are you suicidal or otherwise in need of immediate medical help? She judges that you are short of that, in this case, and takes you through options for therapy – waiting list or private? – and medication. But towards the end of your appointment the doctor frames your situation in a surprising way.

She suggests that what might be happening to you is a kind of crying out for transition, for transformation. Something – or many things – in your life, in your body, your mind and your very soul are desperate for change. This painful, awful moment is a crisis alright, but it is also the birth pains of a new you – a stronger, more balanced, happier and broader version of you. In fact, this is a spiritual crisis, at root, and it will lead, if you take careful and brave steps, towards a life which suits you better; this is the start of a spiritual emergence. Mike Slade's PhD student is setting out to find out whether this approach has better outcomes than our current one, which frames what you are going through in terms of disorders and illness. One sends the message that you are growing, the other that you are falling apart. The question is, which will prove more helpful to your recovery?

'It links to Mad Pride, for example. They are saying,

this is the stuff that makes us human. They don't see these experiences as disorders. Why are we seeking to normalise these human experiences in a way that no one else is expected to? For example, we live with anti-vaxxers. We don't give them treatment! It's not seen as fundamentally not-allowable as a world view!'

The Mad Pride movement grew out of the anti-psychiatry and psychiatric survivors movements; one of its first seeds was *On Our Own: Patient-Controlled Alternatives to the Mental Health System*, by Judi Chamberlin, published in 1978. The title tells the story: networks of people with experience of mental health issues began to question and reject the conventional model, which, they felt, branded sufferers as other, as deficient, as less than normal. Instead, they asserted their difference as in no way 'less'; they began to share and promote the idea that the ways in which they (we!) see and experience the world are valid and valuable. Members of Mad Pride share and campaign for different conceptions of their situations, and for treatments which do not seek, as they see it, to marginalise and devalue them. What is normal? Who gets to delineate and determine it? And what gives anyone dominance over the designation of anyone else? they asked.

The link between Mad Pride and the work of Mike Slade and his colleagues and collaborators is that both groups (campaigners and sufferers on the one side, researchers and clinicians on the other) desire fundamentally to reappraise the assumptions underlying the field of mental health, from the ground up. What if we have misconceived the whole paradigm of the 'well' and the 'ill'? And what if the ways in which we currently believe that those in difficulty should be treated does not optimise their recovery? Starting intellectually and conceptually afresh, how might we reframe people's experiences in ways that contribute, perhaps dramatically, to their healing?

'Does it work for people?' I ask. 'Seeing a breakdown as a spiritual crisis?'

Mike's tone changes slightly, as if the academic, the campaigner and the social scientist in him are in constant flux and dialogue.

'If by *work* you mean, "Is there evidence in the evidence-based empirical medical world?" and, "Has that been obtained by randomised controlled trials?" [the gold standard, as it were, of scientific proof] then, no – that's a different frame of references. Someone walks into a church and invites the congregation to consider the merits of atheism – this is a paradigmatic clash! How do you do a randomised controlled trial on "Supported Spirituality as a Mode of Recovery"? Well you *can*, and it has been done once, and the main finding was that psychiatrists hated every aspect of it. And the reason they hated every minute of it, of course, was they were being asked to countenance and encourage a level of human experience they had neither experience nor expertise nor training in. So no, there isn't that kind of evidence.* On the other hand, what constitutes evidence? And if enough people say something, does that make it evidence-based?'

Mike is wonderfully animated at this point, as we move between hope and **identity**. There seem several different drives here – a sense of injustice, a sense of vast possibility, a sense of an irritatingly flimsy but still entrenched system preventing, slowing or hindering urgent and obvious progress. The orator's power to move, to reveal and convince, blends with the precision of Mike's language and the disciplines of his profession in an unusual way.

'What do people live with?' Mike demands. 'What is their identity? If many people live with very varied experiences of mental health issues, and if they live with varied fundamental understandings of what's going on for them, then

---

* The psychiatrist and author Abraham Verghese, writing in 2008, summed up the historical position: 'The majority position of Psychiatry has been that Psychiatry has nothing to do with religion and spirituality. Religious beliefs and practices have long been thought to have a pathological basis, and psychiatrists over a century have understood them in this light. Religion was considered as a symptom of mental illness. Jean Charcot and Sigmund Freud linked religion with neurosis. *DSM3* portrayed religion negatively by suggesting that religious and spiritual experiences are examples of psychopathology.' Research published in 2015 reported that a systematic meta-analysis of randomised controlled trials on the efficacy of religious and spiritual interventions demonstrated significant effects on the symptoms of general anxiety, and decreased stress, alcoholism and depression.

the idea of telling people, "This is the understanding you should have," is *not* evidence-based. If we tell someone what the "proper", "true" diagnosis is, this immediately precludes other explanatory frameworks.'

The next areas of the CHIME framework are **meaning** and **empowerment**. As we have seen, there may well be times when people who need help find they have to argue with the system which is there to provide it. When, I ask Mike, in order to receive the most suitable and effective kind of attention and treatment, might one reasonably think about not being a 'good' patient?

'When it speaks to empowerment,' Mike says. 'We're doing research in more collectivist societies – empowerment there is not so valued. Here it's like moving from child to adult – it's important that there's some stepping out from the shadow of family. It's important that there's separation from the family of origin, some conflict, some difference emerging, because that's what identity *means*. So it's not being what the powers that be are asking you to be, but being you. That's the metaphorical parallel for someone living with mental health issues – it's not letting that become the engulfing role. It's not letting that become the only thing the person is.

'Because the system isn't very good at that. It often wants that to be the *only* thing the person is. Because a good, compliant patient doesn't have preferences. A good, compliant patient doesn't dislike certain people. A good, compliant patient doesn't say they don't want to

work with particular people, and doesn't have an aspir-
ation to the job that the clinician thinks is too risky.

'And I think those are very important things, and things
a good recovery-supportive system would encourage – as
opposed to the current focus on, *"Take the treatment as prescribed."* There is such a thing as toxic positivity, when life
has treated you badly, or an individual has abused you, or
society has systematically disenfranchised you – it's not
something you should smile through and grow from and
learn from. It's something you should be angry about, and
make a fuss about, and kick back against.'

15. Bouncing back better: Post-traumatic growth

Post-traumatic growth is the most hopeful, inspiring and empowering concept I came across while researching and writing this book. Life itself can be seen as a process of post-traumatic growth, given that things arguably go downhill from the luxuries of the womb, and that difficulties of all kinds, overcome or adapted to, offer potential benefits. The root of the word madness, you will recall, comes from the German 'changed for the worse' – or as we might put it now, traumatised. The notion of trauma as a starting point for growth is a beautiful and beautifully simple concept on the face of it: pain, trauma, hard times, grief, depression, breakdown, harrowing encounters with self-harm, anxiety, psychosis, schizophrenia, mania, eating disorders, addiction, suffering, in sum, can and do lead to people who survive them becoming stronger, wider, wiser, more sensitive – perhaps more fulfilled and more able to help and lead the rest of us. However, in this context, it also turns out to be a field alive with the unexpected. Prepare for surprises. And although we will focus at the more severe end, everything which is covered here does or can apply across the whole spectrum, as we will see, all the way to the most specific and individual conditions.

I ask Mike Slade, Professor of Mental Health Recovery and Social Inclusion at the University of Nottingham, whom we met in the previous chapter, to explain what is meant by, and what happens in, post-traumatic growth.

He jumps to the work of Peter Chadwick – a psychologist and scholar who experienced psychosis, Chadwick is the author of *Schizophrenia: The Positive Perspective*.

'It's the idea that this thing may intrinsically be a *good* thing. It's really very challenging. It conflicts with the world view that schizophrenia is something to be got rid of, to adapt to, to not have dominate your life.

'People have said to me, "It's not like I would have *wished* for this to happen before, but actually the changes that it has produced in me, the growth that it has produced in me, means that I'm really glad it's happened and I wouldn't change it if I had a button."

'And I found that so challenging. So challenging. Digging down into it, the things that are going on there are things like Survivor Mission. So people are saying, "I now actually care, in a way I never knew I could care, about this not happening to somebody else."

'Or people talk about increased compassion – so they say things like, "I used to be really focused on achievement and productivity, and because of what I've been through it's fundamentally changed my relationships with other people. I'm much more compassionate, I'm much more caring, much kinder and more gentle, and I've gained a true understanding that life is hard sometimes." Or it can take place at a more individual level of personal growth – for example, unleashing creativity in the portfolio of things they do.'

Mike's team are at work developing an online intervention to promote positive growth after psychosis, in the form of an app.

'It's about supporting people as they notice and amplify positive changes. It is such a useful thing to consider, and it hasn't ever been considered very much, precisely because of the medical world view that schizophrenia or psychosis are all bad.'

Dear reader, I try not to think of myself as an especially greedy or grasping person, but I hope you will not think less of me if I confess that the mere idea of post-traumatic growth fills me with a delightedly ravenous yearning along the lines of *God yes, I'll have me some of that!* So the question is, does it apply to all kinds of distress, as well as the more severe end? Mike Slade is adamant that it does.

'Growth, rather than reduction, as a result of these types of mental health issues, is not something specific to psychosis. Of course it applies across life experience generally, and to depression and anxiety very much as well.'

'And how do we achieve and support post-traumatic growth?' I ask.

Mike answers in terms of breakdowns, psychosis and schizophrenia, but again, these solutions apply across the spectrum. He does not hesitate.

'Better support for relationships,' he says. 'We tend to

extract people and plonk them in a ward – which in many cases is the worst thing you can do for someone's network. And we need to ask, "What are the protective factors?" We know almost nothing about protective factors – so one of the protective factors for young people is bonds with pro-social peers. Falling in with the right crowd, in other words. So, empirically, health money should actually be spent on skateboard parks, which promote physical activity, and where young people can gather and not be vulnerable.

'To promote more post-traumatic growth, another thing we could do is community-level interventions. So we should bring people together to talk about their experiences – which is why it's so problematic that the voluntary sector is running on fumes. Often volunteers are the very people who bring the community together. The things that often get cut are those softer networks which are so important for individual growth.

'And we need to increase peer support – someone who has lived experience, and grown from it, provides an incredible role model of recovery, but peer support-ers also give practical support. So they might help someone with the confidence to go out, to do things, to go back to the library, to do that thing, whatever it is, that they enjoy. That is about creating virtuous cycles where growth is possible.

'Then we need to look at supporting people going back to work. Actually, supporting people back into employment is a model of how we can support people to grow through and beyond the challenges that they've had. At the moment we push people into the mental health system, which is a ghettoising, separating, *different* identity that just doesn't support the natural processes of recovery that we need.'

Now Mike tells an unexpected story which casts a new light on how we might understand and grow from traumatic experiences. I think it is worth following Mike's teaching on this wide subject, because if you or someone close to you is suffering or has suffered, if you or they have googled it, and if you or they have had contact with health services, the chances are you have encountered what appear to be strong and settled narratives which do not necessarily make sufferers or those close to them feel particularly good about who we are and what we might expect.

But the fact is, these are old, uncertain and developing ways of seeing and understanding distress. The entire field of the mind and its troubles is in momentous flux. A century hence, very little of what you might read on the internet or hear in the culture now will have much sway. So the real point is – let's not wait out our lives, hampered by models which few clinicians believe in anyway, which researchers are questioning and debunking, which manifestly have not worked for huge numbers of people. Let us get on with healing and growing, this year, this month, this week, this day – let us start getting and feeling better *now*.

'When traumas happen,' Mike says, 'like the Grenfell Tower fire, or an earthquake, when something happens and lots of people are affected by a tragedy, what used to happen was that counsellors were parachuted in to help people process the trauma. And so there would be compulsory debriefing for blue light staff, so that they could recount what had happened to them. Weirdly, what came out as a scientific finding – and it changed practice *overnight* – was that the so-called Critical Incident Debriefing is toxic. Not just neutral but *toxic* to natural processes of adaptation and integration and finding meaning in what has happened. And actually, being forced before your time to talk about what had happened to you ended up being less useful than having an available service down the line that you could access if you were having trouble processing it.

'And I think we should learn from that in mental health. How can we support post-traumatic growth? First, we need to give resources that are *available*, not imposed on people. And secondly, easy access to help when the person *wants* it, rather than when, in the judgement of others, they need it. We know that there's something about the person staying in control that actually creates a trajectory towards recovery and finding positive benefits.

'So post-traumatic growth is also about supporting empowerment at every point of contact with the mental health system. Ideally, it starts to take place from when you are at the point of crisis. So you *can* impose solutions on the person – but it's at points of crisis, when the power imbalance is so magnified, that radical interventions have the most power to make changes.'

This all sounds interesting and hopeful but I am not clear what that last paragraph would actually mean or look like, in practice, until Mike tells this story.

'In New Zealand they have the Key We Way National Empowerment Center, a recovery house in Wellington. So there was a traditional psychiatric institution, and they started another one, a peer-run crisis house on the beautiful coastline. People were randomly assigned beds – either to the traditional hospital, or to Key We Way. In the first one they'd be brought in, in cuffs in some cases, and they'd often have a reduced liberty experience throughout their stay.' (I take this to mean the locked wards, the heavy presence of security, the feeling and actuality of enforced detention against your will.) 'In the other, in Key We Way, the first thing that happens is the peer support worker will sit with the person, and not make any demands of them, but instead they tell them *their* story. And the second thing that happens is, they will say, "Do you fancy a walk?" And they will both take their shoes off and walk on the beach. And the trajectory of healing is *entirely* different to the traditional ward. They found there were no risk issues – none of the fights and bullying that were happening all the time on the traditional ward. It just creates a social milieu that leads to wholly different trajectories. And I think we underestimate what's possible, even in times of crisis, if we have a system that provides agency, support and empowering approaches, rather than making demands and requiring compliance.'

Systems change is clearly coming. But how long will it be before mental hospitals everywhere are rethought and renamed as recovery houses? In the final chapter of this book we will see just how varied and effective are different treatments, approaches and ways of thinking that are already available in different parts of the world, and consider what we can learn and lift from them in order to deepen and accelerate recovery and healing here and now.

But if you or someone close to you is in trouble, you need practical and immediate positive steps which can be taken today. Thinking about a friend whose son is at university, where he has been smoking a lot of weed, missing lectures, falling behind and spiralling into feeling miserable, isolated and trapped, I asked Mike for guidance on this common sort of problem. Given all he knows about recovery and post-traumatic growth, what would he advise? I ask him to respond informally, as if over a meal, speaking to a friend; a desperately worried friend. His manner changes, less the professor leading the international research cluster, more the sympathetic fellow parent.

'One of the things is – although it's really hard – the temptation is to get the person to stop the problem behaviour. So, "Can't you see that smoking weed is leading to worsening mental health for you? And can't you see that stopping it will solve your problems?"

'Which is what any loving parent or friend will have in their head. But it is not necessarily a helpful message. Not for that person. The more helpful message is, "You *will* find a way through this. You will find your solution." Because that speaks to a whole different relationship. One of our interventions is called Refocus – we trained mental health professionals to better support the people they were working with in their recovery. The key thing we did was, we trained workers *not* to use traditional clinician–client models, but to use coaching.

'Coaching is based on the assumption that the *coachee* has the solution. It's not the coach's job to *fix* the person: it's the coach's job to help the coachee find the solution that works for them.

'So if I had one bit of advice in that difficult situation, it would be to not be too focused on what to you, as an observer, seems self-evident: "You've got problems because you're doing X. Stop doing X; honestly, it will help you . . ."

'But rather, it's more effective to be focusing on: "How can we help you to find the best way forward? How can we help you to talk to people who have found their way out of the hole that you're in at the moment? How can we help you to have things [in your life] that may help you towards health, rather than feeling you're stuck doing things that are keeping you in this vicious cycle?"

'So *that* kind of agency, that empowerment, that kind of unconditional support, is probably the thing that I'd be suggesting is the most useful contribution of loved ones.'

Rule 22: To help someone who is in trouble, 'I believe you will find your way through this and I am here to help you find it,' is more effective than, 'This is the way to get better.'

Frankly, rule 22 sounds bloody hard to follow. As a parent, step-parent and university tutor (and one who messed himself up with cannabis), the thought and experience of having these conversations makes me deeply anxious, especially if I am to stop myself saying the most obvious thing I will be desperate to say: *For Christ's sake, change your behaviour!*

I really do know how truly, horribly awful is the suffering that dope, depression, anxiety and paranoia can impart. And I feel an overwhelming sense of what Mike referred to above as Survivor Mission: *Please, in the name of all that's holy, don't do what I did, don't continue to suffer as I suffered.*

But I find I trust Mike completely. And never mind me – huge national and international funding bodies and research councils trust and back his work, too. So the next question is, does this approach work for other conditions?

'Is it the same with anxiety?' I ask. 'Is it the same with everything?'

'Yes,' Mike replies. 'You [the person who is suffering] *already* know what to do. Your journey is to find that knowledge. And my contribution is to help that journey. Which is why one of the fundamental shifts is helping health workers to understand that they don't make people recover. *Individuals* do the work of recovery in their own lives. The worker's job is to help that person do that work. And that's a fundamental shift in biomedical ethical expectations. It relieves the duty of care. It's a shift in a way of understanding and relating who has the knowledge, and it changes the balance in that relationship.'

It feels inspiring, even joyful, to hear this. It chimes (sorry) exactly with my own experience. I and my family and our support network came through horrific times to something rich, fortunate and beautiful, and we reached it by intuition, research, trial and error – and it must be said, by the wisdom and efforts of Rebecca Shooter, my beloved ex, who has an extraordinary sense of how families, and post- or patchwork families, can really work. My own progress, from breakdown five years ago to an infinitely, unrecognisably better place now, followed – haphazardly and unwittingly – exactly Mike's formula of Connectedness, Hope, Identity, Meaning and Empowerment.

And so now what I want to know is, how good can recovery get?

Mike smiles. 'You're talking in relation to people who've lived with mental health issues. I think it's nothing to do with mental health. How far can an individual go? What are the limiting factors? All of us have limiting factors. I could never run a sub ten seconds 100 yards. But I don't think there's anything special about mental health that means this is a group that should be singled out to figure out what their potential is.

'For exceptional people the sky's the limit. Look at Stephen Fry and bipolar. Look at Alastair Campbell and depression.' (Both men have made engrossing documentaries about living with their conditions.) 'For most mere mortals like me, you can progress to wherever your dreams and energy and ability will take you. The thing that will get in the way, that we can fix, is stigma and discrimination.

'Stigma and discrimination, *that's* the stuff that, if we're going to put our energy into it – rather than individualising what is a social issue – will make the difference. The better focus for the best minds in the business is, "How can we change society so that people can genuinely fulfil their potential?"

'And you know the big win of that? It doesn't just benefit people with mental health issues. That benefits *all* of us. Which is why, for me, recovery, at its heart, is a social justice issue.

'It's nothing to do with treatment or recovery support or mental health and social care systems – it's a social justice issue. It's about people having a fair go.'

'It sounds as though a lot of this is outside the individual?' I put in. In other words, all this is all very well,

YOUR JOURNEY, YOUR WAY

but how does it apply to us, now, who might be in the midst of an eating disorder, or depression, or a breakdown?

'When the people change, the leaders will follow,' Mike replies. 'I think much of this problem is, often, that we conceptualise it as individual. But it's societal. It's about human rights. So I think if I were talking to an individual I would say, *"Join with others."*

'Because *you'll* benefit, and your wisdom and experience will be of benefit to them. And that helps with the normal need [of any citizen] to be a contributing person, as well as being interdependent and leaning on others. So there are only *wins* for the communities and the networks and the connections that joining with others generates.

'And sometimes it's right to be angry. My passion is based on outrage, it's an emotionally-based groundswell of anger for me, because I've seen that people who are labelled with having mental health issues are not having a fair go. And that's just not on. It's not on, any more than it would be in relation to gender, or ethnicity, or any other aspect of identity.'

'When you say "join with others",' I ask, 'that doesn't necessarily mean spending a lot of time on a Facebook group with other people who have been given the same diagnosis, or does it?'

'It means finding your tribe,' Mike returns. 'Now, your tribe might be diagnostically defined. So it might be, "I live with depression and I joined the Depression

Alliance and I found a very supportive group of like-minded people." That *might* be what it means. But it might be, actually, "I want to change the world and my tribe is other social activists." '

So, in conclusion:

Rule 23: There IS an established and proven route to recovery – it is called the CHIME framework. If you follow it, you will maximise your chances of recovery. If you are helping someone, remember it is not your job to fix them; your job is to support and believe in their power to help themselves.

16. On the ward

If things are too much, if you or someone close to you is breaking down severely, if someone is no longer able to look after themselves, if they need urgent help but they are not receptive to it, if they are a danger to themselves or others, then it is time they were in hospital – either voluntarily, or against their will. For obvious reasons, this chapter will not be much use to anyone in that state when they are in it: during the acute phase of my own breakdown, I was unable to settle down to read or take in anything. So this chapter is for you, their friend, partner, family member or carer, and for you if you feel that in-patient care may be something you need. It lays out what happens in a psychiatric ward, and how you can best help someone who is committed to one. It is an unusual and, I hope, valuable insight, in that very little of what you will be able to find or read elsewhere about life inside a locked ward is written from a patient's perspective.

As we have seen, in order for someone to be detained on a ward a specialist social worker, known as an Approved Mental Health Professional, needs to do an assessment, in the presence of two doctors, one of whom is a psychiatrist, resulting in a form: an order to detain under the Mental Health Act.

Under Section 2 of the Act, you can be detained for up to twenty-eight days; under Section 3 for up to six months – and Section 3 is renewable indefinitely. The doctors fill out a form entitled Medical Recommendation for Admission for Assessment, known as 'Med Recs' in the trade: these two pieces of paper bring into force the powers of the Mental Health Act 1983, and they are serious powers. The sufferer can now be compelled by the police – in some cases, by private security firms contracted by the hospital – to go to the ward.

I went in with a policeman gripping my arm, hard, on the better-safe-than-sorry principle. He didn't want to have to chase me across the car park between the ambulance and the ward, and he was not to know that I was not, then, in the mood for flight (and I was wearing, for reasons which now evade me, my friend's Crocs). One of my friends on the ward told me it took about five police officers to drag him in. Having regained our sanity, neither of us held any grudge against the social workers who sectioned us or the officers who had to take us in. Nor did any of our peers on the ward – the overwhelming emotions on the ward, regarding the people who had dealt with us in our madnesses, were embarrassment and shame.

A young man I interviewed who was admitted to a ward that was at the time terrible, terrifying and disastrously unfit-for-purpose in Broad Green Hospital, Liverpool, told me that he was threatened in the van on the way in by the guards employed by a private security firm: 'You just wait until we get you alone,' one of them said to him. Imagine how horrendous that would be when you were in your right mind, and multiply that by how frightening it would be if you were having a breakdown. It is another reason why I wanted to write this book: people have to know that these wards are a lottery, and though you may have no choice but to participate in sectioning someone – indeed, you may have to fight to get them the care they need – your responsibilities do *not* end here.

If you love someone, or care for them at all, they are relying on you to make sure they are getting proper treatment, not being warehoused in one of the unfit wards which do exist in this country now, where people will be sent today, tonight and tomorrow, and where they are likely to accrue more damage and trauma than that which they were suffering on admission. This assertion is not based on opinions, beliefs or speculations of mine: as we shall see, the fact that dangerously unfit wards exist is known to Approved Mental Health Professionals, psychiatrists, sufferers, families, the press and the Care Quality Commission, which investigates complaints against them. Fortunately, there are simple, vital steps you can take to help someone who is committed to a psychiatric ward.

From the moment you are admitted on to the ward you are the responsibility of the psychiatrist in charge: this person is now your 'responsible clinician'. Although what happens on the ward is in the hands of the ward managers (on mine, the lead manager did admin and had little to do with patients, while the deputy ward manager interacted with the patients and dealt with our needs and requests), what happens to you clinically is down to the responsible clinician, who is a psychiatrist. If you are admitted at night or at the weekend, it is unlikely that either of these people will be present. Instead, the senior nurse in charge will make an assessment and decide on your immediate treatment. In my case, that meant being told to take an antipsychotic and a sleeping pill. I said I did not take sleeping pills, and the nurse said fine, but I must take the antipsychotic. I said I did not want to take it. This put the nurse in a difficult position, and he handled it perfectly. Rather than wield authority, he asked for my help. Although I was as mad as a fruit bat, I was lucid – so when he said, 'Look, it will be much better if you do take it, because otherwise we will have to force you to take it, which will be very distressing for us, and for you, and potentially for the whole ward,' I agreed immediately. (Always, always seek to get alongside the person in trouble, rather than assert your sanity over our distress. Give us as much agency as possible. Recruit us into the service of our own care – it is vastly more effective, fair and humane than coercion. As soon as I realised I could help the nurse and the ward staff by cooperating, I cooperated.)

Some of the older wards still operate a dormitory system. There are about 350 in England. These are outdated and obsolete; the Care Quality Commission has warned that they have no place in patient care in the twenty-first century. As the carer for someone who is being sectioned, this would be the first question I would ask: do they have their own room? If the answer is no, I would take that as a first alarm bell. I would be sure to visit the next day, or at the first possible opportunity, and I would listen carefully to whatever the sufferer told me about their conditions.

You are unlikely to be allowed beyond a visiting area, for reasons of patient privacy et cetera, and your friend or loved one is unlikely to be in a generous, balanced or receptive mood, having just been sectioned, but you need to take what they say seriously. If they are concerned for their safety, or have complaints about their care, you may have to act (see the end of this chapter – 'making a fuss').

The nurse in charge is liable to be someone who went into mental health nursing as a vocation, hoping to spend time with patients and aid in their treatment and recoveries. But due to staff shortages, they are likely to be overworked, rushed, mentally juggling a dozen simultaneous demands, and stressed. In February 2023 the *Nursing Times* reported, 'During 2021-22 some 17,000 staff (17%) left the NHS mental health workforce, up from 13,000 (9%) the year before,' citing figures from the National Audit Office. A mental health nurse told me that teams are spread so thin that one or two people calling in sick or being otherwise unavailable puts the whole ward in a perilous position, and that nurses feel that responsibility keenly. In July 2023 the Public Accounts Committee published a report on the state of mental health staffing. It found 'the percentage of days lost from the workforce due to psychiatric reasons doubled in a decade. NHS England told the PAC that, in common with all NHS staff, mental health problems are one of the biggest drivers of sickness among staff.' Research by the British Medical Association found the reported rate of vacancies in mental health nursing is currently around 18 per cent. But the BMA notes that the actual vacancy rate is bound to be higher: because hospitals cannot afford to hire more staff the jobs are simply not advertised. It seems that around one fifth of this vital workforce is missing.

Those remaining at the front line and those joining it are doubly heroic; it struck me repeatedly on the ward that while my fellow patients and I had to be there, the people who were looking after us came into exactly the same locked ward – with its distressed patients, anxious relatives, claustrophobic corridors and limited natural light – carrying the increased pressure of responsibility, of their own accord, day after day. Take a good look at the people in charge of the person you are worried about. In the best among them you are looking at some of the most remarkable people in the country: people who put themselves in the line of immense stress and pressure, for the thinnest material rewards, simply because they have the extraordinarily admirable calling and ability to help those who need it most. It is worth remembering this. It was only one person's experience of one ward, but what I saw while I was detained was a revolving team of nurses, support workers, caterers and cleaners who were devoting their professional lives to giving expert help, kindness and care.

On my ward, the ward manager had almost no contact with patients, rarely emerging from his office, where he did constant admin; the deputy ward manager was around during the day, but for the rest and the majority of the time we were in the hands of the duty nurse and support workers.

On a good ward, the duty nurse works with huge responsibility, worry and constant anxiety – on a bad one, as undercover documentaries have shown, patients can be neglected or bullied and brutalised into submission, helplessly at the disposal of callous and lazy staff. In 2023, the mental health charity Mind listed recent scandals, including the Essex Partnership University NHS Foundation Trust, 'where more than 2,000 people died over a 21-year period, and misuse of restraint, staff falling asleep and ligature points were exposed'. Then there was the Priory Hospital Cheadle Royal near Stockport, 'where Beth Matthews, 26, Lauren Bridges, 20, and Deseree Fitzpatrick, 30, took their lives.' And Huntercombe Hospital in Maidenhead, 'where there have been more than 1,600 sexual safety incidents in four years.' Huntercombe's name was changed to Taplow Manor; in 2023, the Care Quality Commission judged it unfit for purpose, the NHS stopped referring patients, and the owners, Active Care Group, shut it down. In 2022, the BBC *Panorama* programme secretly filmed scenes of grotesque abuse at the Edenfield unit in Greater Manchester, where staff degraded, assaulted and humiliated patients. Several members of staff were dismissed and the chief executive of the Greater Manchester Mental Health NHS Foundation Trust resigned. Various psychiatric hospitals and units in Birmingham, Liverpool, Newcastle and Manchester have been criticised by the Care Quality Commission, patients' groups, families and the press in recent years.

There is no league table of the best and worst psychiatric wards. Even if there were, families and sufferers have little or no choice about where patients are admitted: the strain on the system is such that you tend to get sent to where the nearest bed is available, and that can be a long way from home.

This sounds bleak because it *is* bleak: a report by NHS Providers, which represents NHS trusts, found that two-thirds of NHS mental health trusts in England are underfunded to the point where they cannot upgrade or repair their facilities. Writing to Members of Parliament in 2022, the then President of the Royal College of Psychiatrists, Dr Adrian James, said, 'Thousands of people with a mental illness in England are being treated in mental health hospitals that are dangerously old and not fit for purpose. Up and down the country psychiatrists are having to assess and treat patients in buildings that are falling apart and crumbling away.'

This is the situation we all face: a mosaic of wards which span a spectrum between excellent and dreadful. But wherever the person you care about finds themselves, there is much you can do to ensure they get the best possible outcome in the circumstances.

On a psychiatric ward, patients are perhaps even more vulnerable than prisoners in jail: less likely to be believed, possibly with fragile senses of self and/or very low or brittle self-confidence; likely medicated; burdened with much experience of not being listened to. In the worst case, your suffering friend or loved one may never need your help, insight and preparedness to make a fuss more than they do while in this supposedly safe place.

If I were the visiting relative, I would take stringent soundings: I would interrogate the sufferer, other patients, other visitors, support workers, the person at reception on the door, the cleaners, everyone, if I had the slightest doubt about the regime on the ward, or any sense at all of something not being right. Remember Juliet Shepherd – don't be British, don't be fobbed off, don't give a damn what anyone thinks. You may be the only person standing between the sufferer and more, avoidable, suffering.

On a well-run, adequately staffed ward with a compassionate and expert team of support workers, nurses and senior clinicians, days tend to follow a simple pattern. Patients, known as 'service users' will have been observed

throughout the night. Different wards have different systems, but on mine someone shone a torch through a
glass panel in the door once an hour, every hour, all
night. Aimed at your eyes, it meant you woke up, or
moved. This proved you were still alive, and the patrol
moved on to the next room. Really good sleep, I found,
was more likely to come in the morning or afternoon, as
a result. In another ward, in a private sector hospital
which I visited for research, managers explained that
they work with patients to come to an agreement over
how often they should be woken with light in the night,
and constantly reviewed the balance of needs between
sleep and safety.

You are woken for breakfast, and you eat under the
observation of the staff. In theory the staff are keeping a
record of your behaviour and any symptoms, which will
in theory be reported to your responsible clinician at
regular meetings.

After breakfast there is the queue for meds. People
lounge around in the corridor until it is their turn to take
their pills. The full staff arrive, including the psychiatrist. In my experience, this person tends to be in a
great hurry. Their presence has a notable effect on everyone: the staff chivvy about looking flustered, and the
patients' anxiety goes up. If you want anything – from a
different dose or drug, to release or therapy – it is up to
the psychiatrist. As your responsible clinician, they hold
total power over you. Thus, major sources of worry are:
will you actually get the meeting with them which you

have been promised, will you be listened to, and will anything change? Psychiatrists are hard-pressed to meet all the demands upon them. When meetings with patients have to be postponed or cancelled, it is very unlikely to be a psychiatrist's fault: in 2021, the Royal College of Psychiatrists reported that there was only one consultant psychiatrist for every 12,567 people. Just one. One obvious reason that 1.5 million people are on NHS waiting lists for mental health treatment is that 10 per cent of consultant psychiatrist posts are empty.

A lot of the patients' time is spent hanging around outside the staff room, waiting for the attention of a nurse or support worker. Waiting for phone calls. Waiting for information. Waiting for packages, for chargers, for replies, for permissions, for response to requests . . . it is – and feels – endless.

For those people not expecting a meeting, most of the mornings were spent watching television or playing pool. There were small exercise yards in my ward – people rarely used them. There was an art room – one person used it – and we once glimpsed the art therapist, in a meeting, but the one session with her that we were promised was cancelled. There were two excellent men who led gym sessions: in two weeks, I had a single one-on-one session (on expensive new equipment, it was pointed out; the ward was new) with a delightful and sympathetic physical trainer, and one session of badminton and football with a handful of other patients and two staff. Both were joyous and tangibly therapeutic occasions, among the best moments of the care I received. My understanding is that this is representative of what happens on most wards. On a ward in Liverpool I visited, there was a gym and a yard; staff said patients had access to them but neither was in use while I was there. On a ward near Nottingham I was given access to the staff but not to patients. On subsequent visits to my ward in Wakefield the situation was exactly as I describe it here.

On good wards, staff make the effort to take patients out on escorted walks in or beyond the grounds, depending on the patients' status; an accompanied visit to a hospital café on site, once, in my case, and a frank and deeply kind conversation. All of these depend on staffing levels, and so are unreliable, but my experience – having been on wards as both a patient and as a journalist interviewing patients – is that good wards make great efforts to deliver on promises and undertakings given to patients, in the knowledge that disappointments in a restricted environment, for people who are effectively prisoners, feel especially painful and humiliating, and are taken hard. Trips out of the ward tend to be undertaken and overseen by support workers, the underpaid, undervalued people who are the backbone of the entire system.

Lunch follows the pattern of breakfast – you eat overseen by staff. The afternoons see many people going back to bed, others whiling away the time on laptops or phones, and visits from family or friends.

While being visited in conventional hospital tends to

feel like being supported and cared for, being visited in a psychiatric hospital can be rather different. Shame and embarrassment are common and natural. While I loved and appreciated being visited by my friends, I behaved like a rude, petulant, horrible sod when my mother made the (prolonged and exhausting) journey from South Wales to West Yorkshire to see me. My behaviour was a consequence of embarrassment at being there, resentment at her insistence that I was in 'the best place' (I was) and general humiliation, I think. Also, once you have said you don't need or want to be there, and that you should be helped to leave, your relative has said you do need to be there, and refused to make the case for your leaving, conversation rather runs out. However, my mother is an astute observer who trusts her instincts. Even relegated to the visiting space, which was the dining room, she could see that the ward was peaceful, the staff friendly and efficient, the facilities modern, the whole place clean and orderly, the other patients not in any undue distress: I was clearly in a safe and caring place. She was therefore reassured, despite my surly insistence that I should be let go, and she returned home feeling that I was in the best place for me (and for my family) at that time. As someone who is supporting a relative or friend, this is the kind of judgement you will have to make. Although I was feeling humiliated and isolated, and ashamed of my predicament, I was not in any danger and not suffering any unreasonable distress. Had I been in real trouble I'd have been a lot more worked up; she would have realised there was something amiss, and acted. So when you go to see someone on a ward, take what they say seriously, compare it with how they seem, and, most importantly, with how the ward looks, feels and sounds, and the state of the other patients.

Although visiting a psychiatric ward is no one's idea of fun, one of my friends, Chris Kenyon, pulled off the exemplary visit. By taking me exactly as he found me, talking to me as an equal, and referring very little to my circumstances, he drew me into a discussion about things he knew interested me. We watched a vote going through parliament that night on his tablet, leading to a comparison and discussion of the story's treatment by different news organisations, wide-ranging political and media chat, and lots of talk about his own doings and plans. 'Use the time to get well,' he said. 'We need you back.' It was beautifully, generously and cleverly done.

Among my peers on the ward, some sat in resentful or awkward silence with their visitors. One was visited by musician friends who brought their instruments, holding gentle jam sessions in the dining room, which seemed a very thoughtful and effective practice – in the time they made music together, they were all equal. Among those who were heavily medicated, there was not much to say, and speech was effortful: but their visitors, often parents, often mothers, were able to keep them company.

If you are visiting, think of ways in which you can

boost the sufferer's senses of self and self-esteem. One of my peers was delighted, one evening, because he was able to help his wife fix their television, remotely, over FaceTime. As he told me about it, he was visibly and obviously proud of himself – 'What's a man?' he asked at the end of the story, rhetorically, with a triumphant flourish. The point is, being under section in a psychiatric ward, for many of us, feels deeply and horribly humiliating. So you could prepare for a visit by thinking about asking for the sufferer's advice, soliciting their opinions, coming up with ideas for any help the sufferer could give with anything, remotely or on discharge, ways in which they are needed or admired. Any boost you can come up with will mean a lot, even if the patient is unable or unwilling to signal that you have helped, at the time.

Other things visitors and friends said to me when I was on the ward, which helped, included: 'These beds are in short supply. This is really expensive care. You are very lucky to have it. Make the most of it.' (As well as being true, it gave my (fairly shattered) sense of self a boost – I was in need and the system was spending time and money on me, trying to help.)

'Use this as a retreat time. Take advantage of not having to worry about anything, or do anything.'

One of my father's friends wrote to me suggesting I start working on a book about what it was like to be sectioned. I felt the same way, and started to keep a diary, which was hugely helpful. I write diaries throughout the winter as the most fundamental, free, private and supportive activity, giving me perspective on the day, writing down things which strike me as beautiful, funny or noteworthy (which makes me look at the world with an eye out for them), and chronicling my miseries as a way of mocking them and myself, getting a hold of them. Putting pains down on paper helps, therapists will tell you. And I can look back at my diaries for the same period the year before, and see that they felt just as awful then, but I came through them.

Perhaps the greatest surprise of finding yourself in a psychiatric ward, whether you went voluntarily, or were compelled to go, in order that you might receive treatment, is that apart from the drugs, there is very little treatment. In the seventeen days I spent on my ward, one trip to the gym and one game of badminton were all the therapeutic interventions I received (apart from the pills). Among my fellow patients, some of the longer-term residents said they had had psychotherapy in the form of CBT. They may not have been a representative sample – I hope they weren't – but they said it was not much use. As one put it, 'I don't need ways of coping with tomorrow, what I need is someone I can talk to about what happened when I was a kid.' Conversations with my peers, and new friends I made among them, one or two chats with support workers, and the wonderful (to the point of game-changing) visits from friends – Doug and Ellie Field, Chris Kenyon and Richard Coles – were the most helpful things that happened to me on the ward.

And I was very lucky to be in with what the staff described as 'a good group of patients'. It could just as easily have been frightening and even more lonely, had I been amongst a less friendly, less warm, less intelligent or more violently troubled cohort. I have been told truly terrible stories of people's experiences on wards, in which psychotic patients were able to access illegal drugs, which made them violently mad.

After hearing one such account, I asked, 'And do you think that sort of thing is still going on now, tonight?'

'I am in no doubt at all that it is,' came the reply.

In my short time there was no mention of my accessing a session with a therapist. I did hear that hydrotherapy was available to some patients in the hospital, and I asked for it (I love a swim) but was told I was not eligible: it was not explained why but I assumed it was because I was not going to be a long-term patient, in the judgement of the staff, and because no clinician had written on my notes that I might benefit from it. As mentioned, there was talk of a visit from the art therapist, but it was cancelled. And that was that. Unless you are very fortunate, it really is going to be you, your fellow patients, and the pills.

The most depressing time of day tended to be the evening meal, when those of us with families would normally be with them, when those who liked a drink would normally have one, when there was nothing to look forward to but the after-dinner meds queue, and another night. Spirits would rise briefly after food, and people would play pool or watch TV. Then came the drift to bed or the solitude of our rooms. The day shift of staff would leave; the night ward rounds would then begin – the torch shining on your face every hour. Often the nights were covered by agency workers: unfamiliar voices and footsteps patrolling the corridors. The feelings of isolation and hopelessness in the nights could be awful – the feeling, which will be familiar to anyone who has spent a night in a police cell – that the world is out there, but you are not good enough, not safe enough or not sane enough to be allowed to be part of it. Night fears in a psychiatric ward have their own peculiar flavours of misery.

The function of the least progressive wards, then, is to warehouse people who are judged a danger to themselves or others, and medicate them until they are either sufficiently recovered to be released, or thought to be effectively beyond help, in which case they are detained under Section 3 of the Mental Health Act and kept inside indefinitely.

Your priority, as someone who cares for someone who is detained on a psychiatric ward is first to be sure they are in a safe environment, and not being further harmed or distressed by a dangerous, chaotic or ill-run ward (see the end of this chapter if they are).

Then, try to contribute as much as possible to boosting and bolstering their sense of self and agency. You can do this by visits, by phone calls, by letters, cards, email or messages, all underlining your faith in them, your certainty that they will come out soon and feel better, and by underlining the good things about being in the ward: you do get a real break (on a good ward), you have time to recover, the stresses and demands of normal life are absent or vastly reduced. In theory, anyone could benefit from having their meals cooked for them, their bed made and their bills, for a short time, paid.

Although I have looked hard at the negatives in this chapter, there are – or can be, and certainly should be – positives. In my case, I felt that being sectioned marked a huge and decisive break between the ways I had been living before the breakdown, and the ways I lived afterwards. One morning – about the fourth of fifth, I woke up, got out of bed, looked out of my locked security window at a bright winter sunrise and said, aloud, 'You are in a mental hospital under Section Two of the Mental Health Act.' It felt like ground zero, the hard rock bottom, as it were, and from that moment I started writing a diary, and beginning to build a new (and, eventually) better, more honest, more balanced, more careful and more grateful life. Being away from the family and relationship stress which contributed to my being there was a boon, and a relief.

Finally, in order to best help your friend or family member under section, think about how you can help them do things differently when they come out.

What changes to pattern, routine or lifestyle can you suggest or arrange? How about radical changes? Two parents I know, recognising that their teenage son was in with a bad crowd and starting to do dangerous druggie things, took him on holiday to the middle of rural France. On the last day they revealed that there were only two return tickets booked, theirs, and informed him that they had arranged a job for him at the guest-house where they had been staying. They would see him, they said, when he had saved up enough to get home. By the time he did, some of the people he had been hanging out with were in desperate drug trouble, and he was grateful he was not among them. I am not suggesting this would be possible or effective in every case – not everyone has the resources for an impromptu, lifesaving holiday – but it is worth trying to give your friend or loved one every chance to make their world after the mental hospital different from their world before, and thinking freely and imaginatively about how that might best be achieved.

Everyone who is detained under section has a right to appeal that detention, and the staff of the ward have a statutory duty to facilitate that appeal. I made clear my desire to appeal on the first night, the night I was taken in. (In fact, I requested a discharge interview and was told there was no psychiatrist available to conduct it. I requested that that person be called at home, as a matter of urgency, and was rebuffed.) The duty nurse assured me he would lodge my appeal at the first opportunity, on Monday morning (it was Saturday night) and so he did.

Once you have stated your intention to appeal your detention, you are provided with a list of approved solicitors who have experience in dealing with mental health appeals. You pick one, they are contacted, and the process begins. Their fees are paid by Legal Aid, so you don't have to be able to afford them.

The firm I picked were excellent. A day or so later, I had a rapid and comprehensive interview with a solicitor who came to the ward and who took comprehensive notes of all my points and recorded our conversation at breakneck speed. I did not know it, but I had effectively set a clock counting down my detention, and all but guaranteed a release, or change of circumstances, within ten days to two weeks.

The reason for this is that a mental health appeal tribunal requires the presence of a chairperson, known as the Tribunal Judge, who is legally qualified, a psychiatrist (but not the one responsible for you) and a lay person with relevant experience. You will be present, as will your solicitor. Your responsible clinician and his or her team on the ward will be required to provide your medical records, their own reports and records on you, and any reports or data concerning you drawn up, held or created by other professionals involved in your detention, such as social workers or Approved Mental Health Professionals. Furthermore, your responsible clinician and possibly other members of the team responsible for you will be required to attend. Although, as it was confided to me by a support worker in my hospital who has seen patients go through them, it is usual for tribunals to err on the side of caution and rule for the continuation of your detention until your responsible clinician determines you are safe to be released, it is not always so.

And whatever the outcome, having to attend a tribunal and justify and defend their decisions places a deal of stress and bother on your responsible clinician, who is in any case constantly pressed for time, and not unstressed by their day-to-day responsibilities.

Thus, no psychiatrist wishes to find themselves at a tribunal, and unless there is absolutely no chance of you winning, and no way of persuading you to drop or postpone your appeal, the responsible clinician will do whatsoever they can to come to an agreement with you, to reach some sort of compromise.

In a situation in which you are effectively completely helpless, the appeal and the threat of the tribunal is the one power you have. Obviously, this next piece of advice can only be of limited use, since most of us, at the time we are taken in, are in a state of disorder and distress – but if you do not want to spend a second longer in hospital than is strictly necessary, I would suggest that you appeal. You can only begin to exercise what little power you possess by lodging your appeal.

Clearly, you do not wish to waste your own, your solicitor's or your ward management's time. After three days of rest, two doses of antipsychotics, another day or two of adjusting to things and generally recovering from the undermining effect of my new circumstances, and I was ready to fight for my liberty. Crucially, my appeal process had already begun. Had it gone to tribunal, by the time the date came up, and given that the support workers said I was 'presenting as sane' within sixty hours of admission, I suspect the judge would have recommended I be moved to Section 17 – a voluntary patient, who is able to begin to prove insight and capacity by making trips into town alone, and home visits. But any solicitor will tell you that any kind of court or tribunal can go either way – as my solicitor said to me, 'I have seen a lot of courts make a lot of bad decisions.'

How your nearest and dearest feel about your state will have a bearing on your situation. My nearest relative – or at least, the person the psychiatrist was investing with that power, my then partner, Rebecca – wanted me to stay in for as long as possible. The break from me, the recent alarm and trauma she had suffered while dealing with my lunacy, and a hope, held by many relatives and carers, that there was some chemical imbalance in my brain which long-term drugs would solve, if only I would take them (and if only it existed), meant that she argued forcefully for my continued detention. Although I wanted to get out as soon as possible, and wished Rebecca would change her mind, I felt it was to the psychiatrist's credit that he took her seriously, consulted her properly, and reported the gist of their conversations to me.

At this point, the psychiatrist is in an interesting position. If they have any reason to suspect you might still be a danger to yourself or others, they have no choice but to prepare to go to the tribunal and seek to have your detention prolonged. The nearest relative may be urging them to continue to detain you – as Rebecca was, in my case. And yet, they want to avoid the appeal if possible. The problem in my case was threefold: I wanted out and appeared sane, the appeal was in progress, and I was refusing to take long-term medication.

So my responsible clinician offered me a deal. If I would agree to take long-term medication and drop the appeal, and as long as I continued to improve, he would move me off Section 2 to Section 17, under which you are a voluntary patient. This would mean I would be allowed out of the hospital, unescorted, first: I would agree to be back by a certain time, but for a few hours I would be free. If this went well, I would then be allowed to go home for a night, and as long as I returned the following day, we would then be looking at discharge.

I took the deal. I was particularly fortunate that I had a flat to go back to, not the family home. It would have been much more difficult for the psychiatrist to discharge me to a residence where I was not wanted, and much more difficult for Rebecca, and harder for me: crisis house workers like Tamara Moon will tell you that the care and respite they give people can turn their spirits and mental state around in as little as a week, but if they then return to the same circumstances that drove them to crisis, the same consequences follow.

Section 17 felt, relatively, a great place to be. Although

the 'voluntary' in this voluntary section is fairly theoretical (if they don't want you to go out, you're not going out), the sense of agency and freedom in just being able to think and say 'I'm a voluntary patient' is a wide world away from how you feel on Section 2 or 3. At the same time, I met patients on the same ward, when I returned to run writing workshops there, who were being moved to Section 17 – the first step to being discharged – against their will. One man did not feel he would be safe back in the world, but the system wanted his bed for someone more ill, and had decided to move him out, step by step.

'You'll be fine,' the support workers told him. He tried to show confidence but it was clear he had none.

I found my first lone, mentally shaky walks into town quite stressful (I'll always have Wakefield), because I was terrified that some mistake or miscalculation might make me late back to the ward and derail my new status. Having to prove you are sane takes it out of you, from eating breakfast in a sane way and conducting yourself sanely on the ward, to coming and going according to set limits.

I figured that although I would have been quite happy to spend the time on the ward in my room, reading, writing and sleeping (I did not have a phone or a laptop that would let me get online), it was wise to show my face in the day room and exercise yards, to interact with the other patients and – crucially – the staff, so that any reports on my behaviour that they might make would support my contention that I was fit to be released.

When I went back to the ward, months later, to run

creative writing classes with the patients, many of them mentioned this – the temptation and the trap that your room becomes. It's somewhere to take refuge, but also somewhere that becomes part of the prison of the suffering mind, a place where you can get into the habit of burying yourself and hiding.

Keep coming out of the room, would be my advice. The support and clinical staff take it as a good sign, as a sign of recovery. I found a window sill on one of the corridors, which had a view and where I could sit and write. There I had lots of small interactions with other patients and staff passing on their rounds. I felt happy and easy there, which made it easy to come across as calm, content and sociable. Playing pool and throwing a ball in the yards gave us some of the best moments on the ward: we were in the moment, relaxed and playful; support workers and patients felt and behaved as equals; we were able to talk easily, partly distracted by the games.

There is much you can take to a ward to improve a patient's experience of detention. Few wards have much in the way of reading material, so books and magazines are helpful. One dear friend sent a copy of a P. G. Wodehouse novel with a note: 'When in doubt – the Master.' If I were ever to go in again I would want the funniest writers: more Wodehouse, plus Joseph Heller's *Catch-22*, Jerome K. Jerome's *Three Men in a Boat*, Stephen Vizinczey's *In Praise of Older Women*, Tibor Fischer's *Under the Frog*, Sue Townsend's *The Secret Diary of Adrian Mole* series and anything by David Sedaris. A good gift might be a beach boules set, as long as the managers are happy it poses no threat. Small luxuries like good soaps, toiletries and cosmetics make a difference. Take clothes and shoes the sufferer would want to have, rather than whatever they ended up with in the rush and trauma of being detained: when friends brought me my own boots, allowing me to discard my mate's Crocs, the boost was enormous; I felt I could take on the world, or at least meet it, without feeling quite so embarrassed.

Making a fuss about detention on dangerous or unsuitable wards

Should your friend or relative who is under section tell you about malpractice, you will have to make a series of judgements. Is it true? Are they so desperate to get out, so generally upset, manic or paranoid that you cannot believe what they say? Are you getting an exaggerated version of the truth? My feeling is that you cannot afford to ignore it, unless it is self-evidently batty. I would take every complaint short of that seriously. Ask to see the ward manager, or the most senior member of staff available, and see how you feel about what you are told. Do *not* be fobbed off, ever. Push harder. Get answers. When appropriate, *demand* action and change.

One young person I know who was horribly abused on a terrible ward said it took him much longer to recover from hospitalisation than it did from his breakdown.

This sort of scandal should never happen, but it has before and it will again. The least we owe our most vulnerable is vigilance.

As we have seen, a patient's power on a ward is limited. You can appeal against your detention, as outlined above. You can register a formal complaint with staff, with the ward manager and with your responsible clinician. You can object to being forced to take a certain medication – if you report a bad reaction you can, in theory, be excused from having to take it, and be prescribed another one instead. (Though I watched a patient make exactly this complaint, and be ignored by the deputy ward manager in the psychiatric hospital where I was treated.)

The most alarming thing I have heard in months of working with teams of Approved Mental Health Professionals came recently, when one said, 'The worst thing is when you do the assessment, and you know you have to detain, and you make out the order, and then someone says, "There's one bed available, and it's at X." And your heart just sinks.' X, the AMHP said, is known to be an awful place, where someone in crisis is likely to be further traumatised, distressed and suffer a worsening of their condition.

If you or someone close to you is detained on such a ward, if things look desperate or in any way unsatisfactory, and if you or they are unhappy about the conditions, or unsatisfied that it is a calm, caring and healing environment, this is what you do.

First, ask to see the ward manager and/or the psychiatrist who is the responsible clinician. Outline your complaint. Request that you (or the person you are worried about) is transferred to another ward.

The chances are that you will be told there is no other bed available, and 'reassured' that the conditions are not as bad as you think they are.

So now you escalate. It should not be difficult to research the board of the NHS trust which runs the hospital. There will be a chair, a senior independent director, a chief executive officer (CEO) and a chief operating officer (COO). There will also be a chief nurse and a chief medical officer (CMO). In my experience, some of these people are likely, at any given time of year, to be on holiday or otherwise absent, and not answering their phones or responding to email. So go for all of them at once. Keep the ward manager and responsible clinician informed of what you are doing, increasing the pressure on them.

Email and phone, explaining in the most simple and forceful terms that the person you care about is not in a safe, caring and healing environment; that they (the trust) are responsible; that you request and require immediate action to rectify the situation; and state that if you are not satisfied you intend to go public with your complaint, and inform the Ombudsman.

Do not be fobbed off with, 'We will look into it,' however earnestly this is said. Say you are not asking for an investigation, you are asking for change. Demand a timeline – by when will your loved one / family member / friend be moved?

There is every reason to suspect you will again be told that there is no bed available, and that conditions are not as bad as you think they are, so now you escalate again. Inform the senior management, the ward manager and responsible clinician that you are taking your complaint to the Parliamentary and Health Service Ombudsman (Millbank Tower, Millbank, London SW1P 4QP. Telephone: 0345 015 4033) and to the Care Quality Commission. Do so. Make your points simply, forcefully and clearly. The hospital management will not be able to ignore this entirely, but they will calculate that your complaint has a good chance of disappearing into a pile of complaints.

And now it is time to reach for the big stick – the one thing that frightens a CEO (of more or less anything, and certainly a hospital) and has the power to put the wind up everyone in the chain, right down to the ward manager who is failing to care for your sufferer and the thuggish nurse or support worker who is mistreating them: bad publicity. Negative reports in the local press. A growing scandal. Horror of horrors – ending up in the *Daily Mail*.

Now, anyone can say, 'I'm going to the press,' and anyone else can shrug that off with a mental, 'Whatever, be my guest,' but there is a cunning and effective way of doing this. I have had to do it, most recently last year, when someone I am close to, who has a specific vulnerability, and thus is eligible for urgent treatment with specific drugs in the event that they catch Covid-19, did indeed catch it, but was simply not getting the drugs they needed and are entitled to. Given that the clock was running, and it was a clear case of incompetence, I escalated immediately through the steps above, stopping short of the Ombudsman and Care Quality Commission, on the grounds that there was no time. My most effective move, after leaving messages and emails for the trust's CEO, COO, CMO and chief nurse was to contact the head of communications – the press office.

Get hold of this person or that office. Outline the problem. Say that you are now going public with your complaint, having received no effective response, tell them you are in touch with journalists, and ask if the CEO would like to make a statement about the dangerous and unsafe conditions on Ward X.

Inform them, and this is a crucial phrase, that you are keeping a 'contemporaneous note', which is a written record, valid in a court of law (you could explain that to them, too). When they thank you for getting in touch and say they will look into it, make sure you have their name (asking for their age adds a neat touch – we want them and everyone else involved to start picturing having to explain to their aunt why they are in the *Daily Mail*) and give them a reasonable deadline, say four hours, before you take their non-response as a 'no comment' or 'did not respond', and go to the press.

When I did this, the following happened: the head of communications (or someone else in the press office) immediately contacted the COO and the CEO, alarmed, asking what was going on. Those people, I assume,

picked up the phone, and – lo and behold, surprise, surprise! – someone was rapidly in touch with the person I
was worried about, saying that the drugs were on their
way. The drugs duly arrived. I am a huge supporter of
the NHS, and I revere its principles, aims and the tens
of thousands of wonderful, dedicated people who work
for it. I am not here to bash it or terrorise its employees.
But if someone I love is in trouble, then I take the atti-
tude that I will get them the help they need, deserve – and
that all taxpayers pay for – by any means necessary.

In order to get this kind of reaction you will have to
be convincing, and the easiest way to be convincing is to
be telling the truth. So look up the local paper covering
the hospital area. It is likely to be a website, possibly
operated by a large national organisation like Reach
PLC, who own swathes of local papers and websites
which used to be local papers. It should be easy to identify the editor or one of the most prominent and active
reporters, and easy to get in touch with them. Call them.
Tell them what is going on. If the ward is dangerous and
unsafe, they will be interested. To help their interest, you
might remind them of the scandal of Edenfield, the
hospital in Prestwich, Manchester, where appalling mistreatment and malpractice were exposed by the BBC
Panorama team. You may well be on the money – there
are many disgraceful wards currently operating. In 2023,
West Lane Hospital in Middlesbrough was found to be
'chaotic and unsafe'; 'abusive' staff subjected patients to
bullying, according to a report commissioned by NHS

YOUR JOURNEY, YOUR WAY

England and independently carried out by Niche Health and Social Care Consulting. Three teenage girls took their own lives there. If you can expose one of these wards, you will be doing a great public service as well as helping the person you are worried about.

Hopefully, your loved one is in a reasonable environment run by good staff who are giving them life-rescuing care. But if you are convinced that your relative, friend or loved one is in a dangerous or chaotic place, and following the steps above has no impact, escalate further. A reporter from a local paper seeking a quote from the hospital about the situation should have some effect, but if it doesn't, or if you cannot get a local journalist interested, you might need to go to the nationals. Contacts for the news desks of all the broadsheet and tabloid papers are easy to find on their websites and on social media. Even more effectively, you could look at the names of the journalists who cover health stories for the big papers and the BBC, and contact them directly. Don't forget programmes like the BBC's *Panorama* and *Dispatches* on Channel 4. No private hospital, no NHS trust or highly placed (and paid) individual in the health-care system will ignore a query from that level of the media.

I do not regard any of this as underhand or unfair on the NHS, and I hope you won't either. The most important duties of a free press are to expose wrongdoing and hold power to account. Journalists cannot do their jobs if they are not tipped off about what is happening to the powerless, and there is no one more powerless than a 'service user' under section in an unfit psychiatric ward.

If all else fails, and you are sure that your loved one is in real trouble due to poor practices, complain to the CQC and the Ombudsman and once you have done that, send me a message via my agents: Rogers, Coleridge and White Ltd, London. I cannot promise to be available to help, but if I can I will, and moreover you can then truthfully tell the ward and the hospital management that they are going to be investigated, and that a journalist has been contacted and is interested. I am asking you, now, to keep records of what is happening on the ward, what you see, hear and are told, and I am asking your loved one / friends to do the same. So you can also tell the hospital management that – remember the phrase: 'We have been asked to keep contemporaneous notes documenting the situation.'

Keep asking them for statements and on-the-record responses. For a newspaper to use what you collect, you will need verbatim quotes, taken down at the time; accurate times and places; an accurate record of who said and did what, where and when; accurate descriptions of anything of significance (which can be eyewitness testimony from people – maybe patients, or other relatives and visitors – who saw or heard things when you were not present).

Essentially, you are building a case, establishing what has been and is happening through a collection of facts, so be methodical and comprehensive. There is space for nuance. For example, a member of the hospital staff might say to a patient, 'Stop making a fuss and go to your room.' But what counts can also be *how* it is said, and the effects of the words. So if the phrase is said with spite, derision and menace, and the patient feels belittled and threatened, that is a very different thing – and a breach of the patient's rights, and a dereliction of the employee's duty of care – from someone saying it gently, kindly or with humour.

Legal and ethical considerations

A psychiatric ward, like all hospitals, is a place where staff and patients have an expectation of and the right to privacy. When I write, publish or broadcast about psychiatric wards, the publishers, producers and their lawyers rightly insist that great care is taken not to identify any individual, except those who have agreed to be identified and/or interviewed on the record.

You cannot simply put into the public domain, 'X is a brute, who mistreats patients and abuses her position of authority, and her useless manager, Y, empowers her.'

To do so would be to libel X and Y – the test of libel is, does it expose the subject to 'hatred, ridicule or contempt'?

The defence against libel is that it is true – but in the UK the burden is on you to prove that it is true, not on X or Y to prove that it isn't.

What do you do? You collect the facts, testimony and witness accounts that show X and Y are brutal, abusive and incompetent; you present your findings to the hospital management, the CQC and the Ombudsman; and you email it to journalists, as above.

And remember, should you have to fight, you can and will win, because you are not going to give up on your loved one, which means that whoever is responsible for the situation is going to crack before you do. People are suffering, now, today, due to a scandalously under-funded system, which has the capacity to do tremendous harm: no one would wish to be in the position of having to take it on, but if that is what has happened to you, adjust to the reality, accept the role and fight like hell.

You are not alone. And you may not feel, at the end of it all, that you have made a great difference. But as a former mental patient, I promise you that even a small improvement in our circumstances can feel like a wonderful change.

17. Healing in action: Art therapy

Researching this guide granted many arresting insights into how we can help people in trouble, and how we can help ourselves. Looking for the clearest, most helpful ways of understanding and addressing painful complexity, and seeking the best ways through it, took me to an unforgettable encounter in Scarborough on a bleak winter morning. In an act of deep generosity and brave trust, a group of therapists and one of their clients invited me to witness and record a session run by Sue Holmes of Art Therapy Yorkshire. Sue and her colleagues first introduced the theory and principles of art therapy, and then allowed me to join a session with a client Sue works with – let's call her Barb.

I want you to know about this because so much of what we hear and read and see of 'mental health' is doused in a grey shroud of misery. The very term 'mental health' feels to me depressing and stigmatising, though I understand that we use it for lack of a better option (though increasing numbers of people, sufferers and clinicians, prefer 'well-being').

But the point is, it does not have to be this way, because the truth is not this way. The truth is, vast numbers of us move to better places, not worse: statistics vary but the National Alliance on Mental Illness in the US puts partial or full recovery from serious mental illness at 65 per cent. The NHS calculates that 49.3 per cent of people suffering from anxiety or depression who completed an NHS IAPT (Improving Access to Psychological Therapies) course recovered from their condition.

The truth is, aside from struggle and effort, the business of healing and recovery is also shot through with huge hope and inspiring progress, and even joy, and laughter. And this is what I found at Art Therapy Yorkshire, in Scarborough.

Sue comes to meet me in the pebble-dash rain at Scarborough station. She is a small, stalwart figure, her hair thick, framing a face with a look I have seen before. You see it in very experienced and expert nursing sisters and exceptional therapists, clinicians and aid workers. It is a look of great in-taking: you feel seen; not judged, but *seen*. Her eyes are large and her expression kind, compassionate, ready for humour or sympathy in a trice.

As we walked down the hill from the station Sue began to tell her own story.

'I was born in New Zealand. And then I got married and we were farming on the North York moors – you know what that's like! Pulling the insides out of ducks. I went to University College Scarborough and did fine art. I became a technician in the School of Education art department. Then at some point we started The Sunday Lunch in Ebenezer Church – people could come in and

have lunch. There were some very vulnerable, very troubled people. It was a free lunch and the police were
amazed it worked so well.'

The police had tabs on many of these people – known
distressed individuals, many living on the street. In other
words, people more traumatised than I was, with fewer
resources, living dangerous and precarious lives – and
just as mad as I was.

'It was not just giving, it was getting something back.
It was hard and joyful work. Lasting relationships were
formed, we made lots of friends, and there were lots of
deaths – some of the people were very ill, coming out of
hospital. We went to lots of funerals.

'To become an art therapist you do a two-year taught
masters, Art Psychotherapy MA. I knew the art stuff –
manipulating stuff becomes second nature. I can do a
good job with most things except for crochet.

'We studied Freud, Jung, where psychoanalysis came
from, the developments after World War One and World
War Two; we learned about the history of the profession in the last fifty years. Along with music therapy and
drama therapy it's the highest and hardest regulated by
the Health Care and Professions Council. We can be
struck off. You have to have done a long placement – I
did mine at a therapeutic centre near York. You do two
and a half years of professional training. If you haven't
shifted your thinking by the end of that, you're not doing
it right!

'You come to a realisation of responsibility. You

thought it might just be nice – people might like to take a bit of paint . . . it ain't like that!

'It comes down to where you want to place yourself. You could set up a studio and charge a lot of money but you'd get a certain sort of clientele. We felt we should be available to all who need it: we felt it should be in our town and not for people who can afford fifty pounds an hour.

'So we decided to form a charity. We got a name, set up a business with no money, no clients and no backers. But if you don't do that, you don't do anything, do you?'

Sue leads me into the Crescent Arts centre, a lovely building, originally the home of the Sitwells. There are paintings all over the walls, there is a café, there are bright galleries, rooms with bean bags and big windows. Other tenants include architects, therapists and organisations working with the disadvantaged.

'WE ARE OUR OWN PROMISED LAND' says a sign.

In the café we are joined by Moyra Bentley and a senior therapist, Peter. Moyra is the Chair of Art Therapy Yorkshire; Peter leads Art Therapy in Education and Looked After Children.

'What sort of people do you work with?' I ask them.

'Very vulnerable people are our main client base,' says Sue. 'There's a lot of abuse, neglect, abandonment and grief.'

Peter is a strikingly gentle man, quiet, who looks at you thoughtfully through his glasses. His is an unobtrusive presence but when he starts to talk to you his focus is carefully, kindly intense. All three have this quality of seeing, of holding a careful space in the way they are with you. I ask Peter how it works.

'We have to start somewhere,' Peter says. 'The initial ten sessions give us the chance hopefully to resolve an issue, but it's just as likely those ten sessions are an assessment in which we work out an objective and an aim. What issues we can do something about, and their [the client's] and our objectives, and our aims.

'Often people are socially isolated with low self-esteem. Pretty well everyone we work with has low self-esteem. First we try to use the fact that they're coming out, they've come to the space, they're looking for help; it's about recognising they've started their journey. That works on self-esteem and confidence. They're now out and moving in the community. What happens is we take on this initial issue – depression, anxiety – and we address that: now they're leaving the house, they're out and doing, and then the other boxes begin to be unlocked. So then we can work on whatever it is – abuse in childhood, neglect or self-harm.'

'We've got to start the exchange,' Moyra says, 'and then we can make a very productive difference. Ninety-five per cent of the people we see say they see a positive difference.'

Sue leans forward. 'We talk about resilience; something that would have floored them no longer makes them self-harm. So we say, "You were drinking yourself to oblivion – you were heading for hospital – look how far you've come!"'

The building up of the self, through the identification and celebration of progress, is fundamental, they say. Now Peter becomes markedly animated. His body language is clear and excited: this *works*.

He says, 'Acknowledgement of progress is a *major* part of what we do. A lot of our progress is in the availability of the creative medium. It might be art materials or going for a walk, singing, dance – finding something within each person – a creative way of dealing with their issues. Something that means they've just been able to *think differently*.'

'It's a what-if-something possibility – because it's a liminal space, the arena of creativity,' Sue puts in.

I ask, naively, if this means that their clients are making art directly about what is troubling them.

'Well, the process of recognising what your narrative is may or may not manifest as a painting or a model,' Peter says. 'But it invariably does manifest. Just not as a figurative or descriptive piece of art.'

'The narrative is theirs,' Sue emphasises. 'It's their story. We're witnesses. Guides and witnesses. We can see or say something about their story they won't have said before.'

I ask them to take me through the structure of a session. We will see this happen, later, with Barb.

The first five to ten minutes of the session, Peter says, are about what's been happening: 'How are you?', 'Are you eating and sleeping?' Therapist and client chat while they select the materials.

'Sometimes they might discuss a previous painting,' Sue says. 'It depends on the relationship.'

Then the work begins. Around ten to fifteen minutes from the end, while putting the materials away, there comes the opportunity to reflect on that session. The client is invited to speak, perhaps more broadly, about thoughts and feelings, insights or issues that have arisen during the making.

'Does it make a difference if you are good at art?' I ask, mindful that I have not done any since I last painted a watercolour when I was about thirteen.

Sue shakes her head. 'People who have done art can get stuck. People who've not done it since primary school can be very surprised and make something beautiful. We can buy different materials. One young woman had a beautiful touch – she made something 3D – melted and dribbled – it looked like potato chips – we had belly laughs! And as they are making, I might offer into the space some reflection. Some of our clients are non-verbal.'

The strangest thing: as the three of them sit around a small table in the small café on this dreary day, having fought and fought for the funding, the recognition, the space, the time, the opportunity to help, I feel I am in the presence of greatness. It is a greatness that walks unseen among us, all the time. This is a greatness that receives almost no wider or political recognition, which makes nobody wealthy, which requires a defiant gift of energy and determined giving, and an endless fight against inertia and obdurate structures. It is a gift that is life-enhancing, and it is visible in the lines around Moyra's eyes – the burden of the administrative, constructing and maintaining battles has taxed all three of them, but fallen particularly on her as Chair, I suspect. It is in Sue's quality of complete attention, and in Peter's emphasis and gaze as he speaks.

'It's about allowing space for them to come to us,' he says. 'Not pushing them. We ask therapeutic questions, of course, but the beauty is the table, the art, art as a kind of person, an intermediary. The art-making process resolves the tension. Clearly, we want the client to come to us, but sometimes we just gently nudge. Some people pour out their whole life story. We don't necessarily invite it: we want to be able to help but we don't want to open the whole raft of issues and then not be able to deal with them. There has to be a dialogue about aims. If someone's been abused, their life ruined, they've attempted suicide, what can we change in this period?

'What we can change is the viewpoint – that back-story has ruined or messed up your life *up to this point*. How do we get to a different horizon? What do you do now – you've been staying in? We find what it is that the client is able to do. Photography. Painting. We try to find their way of seeing differently and their sense that they are worth something. Most have such a low sense of self-worth. That's our job – flipping that perception of what they are *worth*. To do that, you have to have some-where to stand.'

He sits back and pauses. 'After ten or twenty weeks we review. If we've got funding for twenty weeks. It's not about having something at the end! It's allowing yourself to explore yourself. *You're* the artwork!'

Moyra and Sue agree strongly.

Peter says, quickly, 'People are always pushed to be better. They are continually set up to fail. They are always striving for a moving target. But you can think differently. Recovery starts with perspective.'

The person we are going to meet is somatic, Sue explains – her experiences manifest especially strongly in her body. 'Her family explodes, her appendix explodes,' Sue says.

We meet in the lobby. Barb is a charismatic person, loquacious, warm and outwardly jolly.

We go up to Sue's room, an art studio and office com-bined. Pots of brushes, paints, work on the walls, stacked shelves and crammed cabinets, hundreds of small objects and flocks of pens and pencils are too much kit to take in, but they are all herded into their type and area, martialled like ranks of keen runners, kept behind their particular starting lines, leaving the space and the table free.

Sue unfurls a large piece on the table, a dark crimson semi-circular sun, torn and beribboned. She and Barb discuss it.

'You did it with whole-body movements,' Sue says, and she mimes the memory, swinging her hand and torso over the table, over the piece.

'It would look like menstrual blood to someone else!' laughs Barb.

'This bottom corner is interesting,' Sue says, 'There's something dark here . . .'

Barb runs her hands over the work, seeming to remember. She is smiling, at the memory of the doing, rather than the subject, I think.

To me Sue says, 'This space gives me permission to ask, and this –' she gestures to the painting – 'this stays in this space. The work stays here, it's private and it's generally not viewed by anyone else.'

Barb talks about her body, about needing space, about her family, about a traumatic party that she threw in the hope of making everything better, which blew up.

Sue gets out pieces of another of Barb's works, a ceramic sculpture, and they laugh as they try to fit it together.

'It's a lady garden!' Barb cries, delightedly amused. 'I didn't know it was until I'd made it!'

And now she speaks, moving the glazed and fractured pieces around, like a lumpy jigsaw which will never quite join up.

'Mum would say very hurtful things. At the party I wasn't well, I should have stayed in bed. She said, "I know you've never wanted me to be your mother." Dad walked off. I just stood there. I thought, "If that's what you've always thought from birth . . ." I spent the first ten weeks of my life in a ward with her while they were treating her. I've detached from myself going through it – but if I write it or paint it or express it through art, I'm able to feel the feelings I'm shut off from. If someone needs me, I'm there. But I can't see that unless I look back at it through art. That's how I found the strength to leave my dad – who I thought was my protector.'

Sue moves the clay pieces towards her and Barb shifts them around. She is smiling now.

'Take a lump of clay and something happens. I worked this clay, it was a whole-body experience. It had the form of a pelvis. Bits came down into the V – and that's the bejewelled piece. I was focusing on the moment, on a very small person, on glittery leaves . . .'

Sue joins in. 'You started laughing, and then you came up with the phrase, "It's a lady garden!" There was this deep pool which, to me, is the thing that appears in the corner of the other pieces. There's this jewelled piece with the explosion in the corner . . .'

Barb says, thoughtfully, 'The piece I did yesterday when I was worrying about my relationship, all relationships, and worrying about who I was going to lose next.'

Sue is constantly moving the pieces and reflecting on Barb's work.

'And then you chose this piece,' she said, 'and made it beautiful.'

Barb laughs. 'When I'm having a bad week I email Sue and say, "Get the red ink out!"'

'Look at the range of shift and movement,' Sue says, meditatively.

As Barb tells a story about stress making her ill, Sue is in motion, packing away and unpacking pieces of art, getting out different pictures, displaying them for Barb to look at as she continues to talk. She had a cyst which completely vanished, without surgery – unheard of, according to her doctor.

Barb ascribes it to what has been happening here. 'It was a very strong crossroads moment. What would have happened if I had not worked through things here?'

'I can't make that claim,' says Sue.

But Barb is in no doubt. 'We always have things, and things we go through have a very physical effect,' she says.

I think Sue is floating different options of materials and approaches past Barb, without saying explicitly that this is what she is doing. I think many offers are being made here, without the language which would force Barb to accept or reject them. Sue produces a box of cuttings and postcards.

'I like to work with collage,' Sue says. 'Different thoughts will lead to different things. I think it's a very powerful shortcut. My collage box is curated – lots of fine art things. These artists all looked at life, at human-ity's experiences. I don't use papers or magazines – they're triggering. These have all been mediated through the eye and hand – they're ways of using human experience. I work with Miró, with Gaudí, postcards . . .'

Now she produces a collage of Barb's, dark tonal mixtures of blues and greys, part of a submarine, part of a town horizon, a church. As she looks at it Barb talks about a pathway and a bench, a bench which was very significant to her, where she had a conversation with her father which changed everything between them. This collage, which she made while thinking about it, she says, helped her find a pathway between the bench and here.

As she talks Sue watches her closely. 'How do you feel?' she says, suddenly.

The collage, with the sinister images of the submarine and dark church, is clearly hugely powerful for Barb. It has an eerie quality that I also feel. I can see it now, feel it, as I write.

'I feel cold,' Barb says. She sits down. She tells a long story of her family troubles. At the end, she pauses and says, 'I think I know enough.'

Sue says, 'I think so too.'

We agree to take a break and not talk about anything at all.

When we return, the session proper begins.

Barb describes the traumatic conversation with her father on the bench. She made a sculpture with a caption: 'We sat, I left.' But talking about it now, she says, she realises it should be: 'We sat, I'm left.' She describes a road between past struggles – and losing people along the road – and present safety. 'Where someone cares,' she says, looking at Sue.

Today she is going to make a piece of work about a journey, a terrifying night journey during which she was urgently needed in different places, on a night of dark and deadly traffic, on a road with no stopping places, when terrible news and ceaseless demands were coming from her phone.

Sue produces paper. Barb chooses two large sheets of black, and a paint colour, Prussian blue.

'My favourite colour!' says Sue.

Beautiful old brushes appear, found at a car boot sale. They chat as Barb makes a road like a meandering river of Prussian blue across the wide black paper. This is the road she travelled that night. She draws a bright red square, squiggled on by hand, and works liquid black paint marks into the surface as she describes looking for a safe place to stop during the rush hour, and a crisis phone call with her mother. And they talk about that night, that journey, as Barb rubs the paint in.

Sue appears to be fiddling around, moving things closer, facilitating almost like a technician, while Barb is entirely free in the space, talking and painting. But sometimes Sue stops the flow and intervenes.

'You know you *are* a kind person, don't you?' she says.

At the time, I thought Sue was offering immense empathy. But on reflection, I think it was principally compassion – feeling *with* Barb even more than feeling *for* her. She switches the perspective in this way – from being *in* the journey to being at a vantage point *over* it. And she joins Barb in the places she describes.

'I was looking for a place to be sick,' Barb says.

'What do you think the sickness was?' Sue asks.

Barb is painting in royal blue, a safe place off the road.

'I think it was the sadness,' she says, and she recalls the details of the road, the night, the journey.

Sue agrees. 'Yes, the road is very fast just there, the hill is very steep . . .'

Barb describes being sick in her hands in the car and the core-deep noise that came out of her. 'I just started to scream and howl . . .'

She talks about the strange feelings and effects of the sickness, the wailing. The scenes are so vivid for her, and so fluently described, that Sue and I might as well be there too, in the car, in the panic and fear and despair.

At the end, after a pause, Barb says, 'Admittedly it [being sick, and the scream] got me to a point where I could drive back safely.'

Sue says, softly, 'It's such a significant moment. Something has left you, physically.'

Barb says, 'It needed to come out.'

Sue says, 'It came from your core, almost? It was your core?'

The changes in register are astonishing, the conversation so trusting and tenderly navigated. One moment Barb is in the worst places, the next she is here, and all the time they are both able to talk lightly, too, and often laughingly about such pain. Barb's hands are happily covered in paint. She talks continuously, going into details of the night, the route, the phone calls, the feelings.

Sue says, looking at the paper, 'It's often the arche-
typal that comes out.'

Barb replies, laughing, 'That's why it's that sticky blue,
because it [the situation with her family] still looks shit!'

They study the piece, the map Barb has made, looking
for a safe place.

'I don't think it's here,' Barb says, pointing at her house.

Sue says, 'But it could be a stopping place? A safe
place for now?'

'Yes.'

'So that's a lot. And it's a lot for one day.'

They are both looking at the piece. There is a reflect-
ive stillness which seems to have come the way the
ending to a good story comes, naturally, in the right
place, time and atmosphere.

'We haven't talked about this before, this journey,' Sue
says.

'No.'

Barb looks absolutely in the moment as she describes
conversations she had that night – which might be taking
place there, in the picture on the table in front of her –
and how they hurt her. They are right there.

At one point Sue takes her hand. 'Are you cold?'

'Yes. Goosebumps. But I'm fine.'

Afterwards, Barb says, 'I know the level of trauma
now. I didn't know the level I had in me before we started.'

She tells Sue that Sue has carried her, saved her in
many ways, and through her, saved her child too.

*

The time was up and Barb left. She was different from when she arrived.

At the start she was all nervous energy, her gaze and focus downward, a-jangle with bubbles of nervous laughter, unsettled. My presence was part of that, but I think only a small part; she was palpably carrying more when she arrived than when she left. She smiled throughout, but they were quieter smiles now; she seemed to have released something, set down something.

The pieces they started with, the clay and the collage, were a way of recapping the work they had done, the moments of trauma they had addressed, and a means of reconnecting with Barb's story, as she had told it to Sue, up to that point.

Sue did not tell Barb which part of her story to work on next; it seemed to arise organically. By setting it down together, Sue providing the materials and the gently prompting questions, they seemed to be able to address it side by side, and to pour its pain and trauma into the painting. Had they been sitting facing each other, as in a session of talking therapy, the story of that night would have been incorporeal – real in Barb's mind and memory, and imaginatively constructed in Sue's thoughts, drawn from whatever Barb was able to remember and describe. In some way, I felt, it would have remained there, in the air: Barb would have told it, and Sue heard it and questioned it, both drawing whatever they could from the words, from the account. Sue could have looked for the positives in it – Barb's strength, her care, her resilience, her eventual success in making it safely home. Sue could have validated Barb's feelings and empathised with the experience.

But the difference between that and what they actually achieved is what struck me so powerfully. Working side by side they seemed able to move fluidly between the events of that night drive, Barb's memories and reflections, Sue's empathy and understanding, and the painting itself. Somehow the making of the work allowed the events and consequences of that awful night to be drawn out, and worked into the creation of the piece, but also to be set down, to be placed in proportion, to be seen literally from above and emotionally from a balanced distance. It was extraordinary to witness; it felt as though they were making something sacred or occult, something invested with the power of holding pain and trauma, an artefact with the power to draw these forces out of Barb and to hold them.

Barb was palpably more free and much lighter when the work was done, as though some cluster of pain and trauma had been lanced and dressed. At least some – perhaps much – of the distress of that ghastly night and all it meant to Barb is not in her, now. It is on a large rectangle of black paper and a river of Prussian blue, safely locked away in an office in Scarborough.

The legacy of that astonishing day has stayed with me. If you can possibly access art therapy, I cannot recommend it highly enough, obviously. If you can find art classes of any kind, there is no reason to let inexperience or doubts stop you going along. Statistics – the quantitative measure of these powerful, qualitative experiences – as ever, vary, but studies in the US found that art therapy improved symptoms, raised self-esteem and improved social behaviour among dementia patients; in healthy volunteers whose stress levels were measured by cortisol levels, 75 per cent saw a drop between the start and the end of a session. At Drexel University in the US, researchers found that drawing, colouring and doodling, measured by functional magnetic resonance imaging of the subjects' brains, showed that all three activities increased blood flow in the medial prefrontal cortex – a part of the brain's reward pathway which makes you feel good, or better.

Among people I know who make art, every one of them benefits, whatever they make. One friend, who has suffered burnout and other trials, and who lives alone, paints and draws. Some of the work is resonant, and she keeps it. Other times, she sits down to it knowing that the work is not the point, but the making of it. 'I'll just scratch around and tear it all up,' she said, laughing. It is as much a part of her well-being as cycling, going to the gym, walking and meeting friends.

My mother, who lives alone in Wales, has constructed, without consciously meaning to, a life strikingly rich in well-being. She looks after a flock of sheep, tends to the plants in the garden, maintains a regular schedule with the bird feeder (saving every penny on her own costs in order to keep her animals fed and cared for, and the birds fed), which means the garden is busy with chaffinches, yellowhammers, dunnocks, tits, a pair of collared doves, bullfinches, and a rook who seems to have adopted the place, and her. Painting watercolours at the kitchen table and making ceramics when she can are among her greatest pleasures.

My ex goes through bursts of making – one year she folded magazines and old books into ornaments; another year it was glass and tiles; last year she and our son gathered broken crockery from somewhere and reconstructed it with gold paint and glue in the kintsugi style. Her absorption and tranquillity in these moments is truly beautiful; an atmosphere of peaceful concentration seems to spread through the whole house, the whole day.

I asked Sue if it is possible to be your own art therapist; she said you really need someone trained in order to get the full effect. Art therapists are trained in psychodynamic therapy, psychoanalytical theory, clinical work and contemporary art practice. But the act of making – in your own company or the company of others – is intensely therapeutic. We are not machines for turning time into money; since our earliest ancestors we have deepened our days and given meaning to our lives and times through the expression of our thoughts and feelings in painting, carving, sculpture, storytelling and music. One of the eeriest sounds I have heard was the wuthering, whirring song of a carved wooden lozenge on the end of a strip-rope of animal hide, whirled around and around, creating the music archaeologists believe our ancestors made.

The cave dwellers of the Dordogne valley painted bison, horses, aurochs, rhinos, big cats, deer and bears and ibex, and a man with a bird's head. The bridge between the figurative and the abstract, between the painters then and the viewer now, between all we see and all we dream, is traced out in reds, browns and ochres, golds and black. The paintings dissolve time – 17,000 years disappear as you stand there. (The oldest cave paintings so far discovered, in Indonesia, are thought to have been made 40,000 years ago.) The experiences of being alive, of being, of doing, of feeling, of fearing and loving, of hunting and fleeing are all there. The act of answering the world and what it makes us feel, with a world made in pigment, is there: not so much represented or recorded as *enacted*. In some very strong, strange way you feel they were not made in the past. They are made now, in the instant that you see and feel and hear them. Take a piece of material, they say. Make a mark. There. See? There was nothing, now there is something – there is something made, and there is a maker. There is you.

The insight into the links between the body, the mind and what they make together, whether that is a scream, an uprush of nausea or a painting, was so strong and so obvious in that session with Sue and Barb. Just watching them and listening to them, hearing their laughter (the encounter was astonishingly lit by it) and feeling the meditative calm with which they were able to defuse such fear and hardship – defuse and transform and do something with it – seemed to settle something in me.

If I have been questing, throughout this guide, to find tangible proof of all the theory, the ideas, the stories and the to-the-best-of-our-knowledge that these chapters contain, I found them there. Talking and sharing; listening and being listened to; making and doing: these *really work*, and they really are available, in degree or in abundance, to all of us.

18. How to talk to someone in trouble

It would be a rare life now that did not involve talking to someone in difficulty, someone whom you want to help: how do you do that best? This chapter is about how you communicate with someone in trouble – including, perhaps, with yourself.

Many people have a particular gift for listening, for giving reassurance, for bringing a degree of light and hope, for prompting insight, and among those people, some have it in extraordinary abundance. Our guide is John Mitchell. Until recently, John led and managed an AMHP team in the south of England. When someone might need to be detained ('sectioned') in a psychiatric ward, an Approved Mental Health Professional is the person with the final say; they undertake a Mental Health Act assessment, and if they do not agree to detention it does not go ahead.

It is a demanding, stressful and crucial role. Often, AMHPs find themselves balancing risk to the sufferer with a duty to avoid detention wherever possible. In the community of specialist social workers who deal with mental health, and in the wider field of psychiatry, John is an innovator – an expert and successful professional whose ideas, approach and training are influencing a generation of his colleagues. John knows the field from both sides. His own journey has seen him detained in hospital several times.

We had worked together online but I had not met him until a cold and sparkling winter morning in Milton Keynes, where he collected me from the station.

John might be a businessman working to his own timetable: there is something carefully, professionally put together about him. His face is lined and smiling, his gaze wry and penetrating, the eyes a pale bright blue. As he drives me to his home, I ask John how he came to his profession.

'I saw AMHPs at work and I thought, "I could bring something to this role." Some were frightened of the job, and some were comfortable with it. I read the textbooks as a detained patient. The humour of it all, however dark – perhaps very dark! – is what you need to survive, both as a patient and a professional. You know how you could tell the difference between staff and patients on a ward? The patients looked at you. The staff didn't, because they didn't want to meet your needs. They tend to be rushing to fulfil the demands on them. I went on to manage an AMHP service. I've been working in it for just over twenty-two years.'

Before asking about how we as lay persons might approach and address our loved one or friend in trouble, I enquire about John's professional approach. From his work at the most demanding end of the spectrum, where he is peerless, John has much to teach about how we can be of most use, and about how people in trouble can and should be treated by specialists and services. We began with the basics he considers when dealing with someone in crisis.

'People in crisis don't tend to fear *you*. They fear what's going on. You can only calm them if you aren't afraid yourself. Many professionals are highly anxious – "What happens if I get this wrong?" That happens with suicide risk in particular. We detain comparatively few people because of risk to others, although that changes in the inner cities – the dynamics of an area change the dynamics of assessment. And the spectre of the coroner may haunt our imaginations, in ways that lead to unhelpful, risk-averse detentions.

'When you get a referral you need to think, "Who *is* this person?" If it's someone who has been in the system for years you will often look in vain for the *person* in the notes. You'll think, "They need so much quetiapine et cetera, and a dose of something else." *That's* who they seem to be. But it's not. It's about seeing the question that needs to be asked. What can the person tell me about themselves? Who is there in the family, or a third party, who's known them for a period? Confidentiality limits what I can tell you, but not what you can tell me.

'I often try to see the person with no doctors present. I explain what's going on and find out where that person *is*, psychologically. Offer an open mind, take that person as they are. I try to avoid set patterns. Many doctors have Mental State Examination questions in mind. Although relevant, I don't want to see those questions dominate the encounter. I might ask, "What most worries you?" "Why have the police brought you in?" "Why are we here?" "Tell me the story from your point of view." "What needs to happen now you are here?"'

In more severe cases, especially involving delusions or what is known as a 'florid state' – if someone is talking too fast, having flights of ideas – John takes a particular approach.

'When someone has elevated mood they have pressure of speech, they jump from topic to topic, they may be grandiose. And I know I'm not going to get many chances to say anything. So I need to offer more chances to the person to explain before I win the right to ask a question. Someone with elevated mood may give you very little time to prove you are worth talking to. Are you authentic or inauthentic? Even the way you sit down, even your first question – "Would you like a cup of tea?" – are vital. Bipolar, depressed, dementia, personality disorder – they are all only archetypes, and not very helpful ones at that. Some people will be expansive in a friendly way, some will be irritable. More will be fearful or apprehensive.

'The essential thing is giving the person the chance, and being tolerant of something that appears to go nowhere; and the more people who are there – doctors, police – the more the system's clock is ticking. I try to generate the illusion that I've got all the time in the world for you. I have the notion of, "Can I be helpful?" not, "I must be helpful." It's about the possibility of helping, particularly in finding ways to avoid detention, not, "I must come up with the answer." Of course, in my job, sometimes the answer has to be detention.'

So what – or whom – does the person in trouble really need?

'What the person needs is someone extraordinarily *ordinary*, someone who accepts your suicidal thoughts, who can get alongside you. It's not knowledge that you need so much as a determination to find the humanity in whoever this person is. The difficulty for professionals is feeling that we've got to accomplish a series of set tasks. This can leave the person we're assessing feeling incidental to a professional process: "I've got to *do* – I've got to *do* antipsychotics, I've got to *do* a care plan." And quite often the person wants more of you than they can have – more time, more attention.

'And as an AMHP you've got a role in mediating society's need for social control. So you need to assess yourself first, then the psychiatrist you are working with, then the service user.

'So, for example, a psychiatrist who is an expert in dementia may not necessarily be the best person for a traumatised nineteen-year-old young woman. We need to manage psychiatry so that it benefits rather than unnecessarily antagonises a person at risk of losing their liberty. It can be an AMHP decision – do we break down the door, and potentially traumatise this person for life, or leave them suffering? It can be an all-or-nothing decision.

'Suppose it's someone with a persistent delusional disorder – "the neighbours are monitoring me". But look at the totality of beliefs and behaviour: I can still function, I can go shopping. Someone with that condition often won't respond very effectively to medication, so if you detain you are just warehousing them. So we've got to think, what purpose will hospital serve? Is there any alternative? Is there a possibility that in hospital this person might get worse?

'So suppose the Community Psychiatric Nurse comes to see you – you don't like the medication they give you but the CPN *listens* to you – so there is a balance of benefits for *you* that might look quite different to a professional's perspective. Perhaps the drug isn't going to show you the way back to normality – it might be the face of the CPN listening to you and taking you seriously that's showing you the way back.

'Say someone makes a very serious suicide attempt, they're in hospital, their mental state doesn't fit any category, their suicidality is strong. We will communicate our anxiety to you, and you will see that. You feel like a scary person, or alienated. And some people find it more invalidating *not* to be detained. But if you think I might be genuine, if my anxiety isn't catching, then we have a chance.'

To give an example of how best practice can work, John tells a story.

'A young man of Chinese heritage is not giving details of his identity. I shall call him Peter – he had another anglicised name. He's been brought in by the police from a bridge where he appeared likely to jump. An assessment has already taken place. Two doctors have made medical recommendations for detention. The AMHP would have detained, but there was no bed for the admission, so she was legally unable to do so, and is now unavailable. Those professionals are worried, not so much by mental illness as by Peter's actions and apparently uncooperative attitude. It might seem that they felt the need to detain him almost as a punishment for not giving his details. They have legally adequate reasons in writing, but few real explanations. Where is his suicidality coming from? Peter's telling them virtually nothing. Two days later, he's still sat in the lounge of the "place of safety" with a TV.

'I take care about the way I enter, not wanting to appear that I own the little space he has. I sit down, at a little distance, alongside Peter, notice his tea is nearly finished. He doesn't have to look at me if he doesn't want to. If we're opposite each other, we have to make or evade eye contact. I'm trying to get into his mind – how does it feel to be in my presence? I'm trying too to act in a culturally sensitive way.

'I'm trying to feel where you are least uncomfortable, and work with that. If I'm next to you I can go back to my days of being a patient with you. I can find the optimum place to give you my time. I'm trying to slow *everything*.

'I speak slowly and softly, sending a message – I'm not going away. Something like, "The guys you saw yesterday were really concerned. This is why. What do you think about all that?" Then I talk briefly about my uncertainty. "Should I detain you? That doesn't feel quite right, but I'm going to need your help to unstitch this and find out where we can go." I'm taking it so slowly. Eventually, Peter tells me about his perfectionism, his troubles with university, his father, his parents. I take the trouble to remember the details – the name of his sister, their dog's name – he may think, "Oh, perhaps someone is taking notice of *me*, not just my suicidality."

'Peter tells me about his dad, how he doesn't understand. I try to put myself in the position of being his dad. I say, "We should call him, but you're going to speak first."

'We built something that allowed that conversation, and his dad gladly travelled a hundred miles to the place of safety and took him home. I talked to the team where he lived and said, "He's not that suicidal. He's shocked by how suicidal he was yesterday. He doesn't need to be in hospital."'

John pauses and smiles slowly.

'There's no magic in it, but you're trying to do something both ordinary and magical. I can only do this by reminding myself what it is like to be interviewed with your liberty on the line. You need to be able to imagine this if you are to create the space for someone to trust you against all odds. Professionals don't realise *they're* being interviewed.'

*

John's next story is from the extreme edge, but I think it is worth hearing for its implications: this is about how far listening and connection can take you into the world of someone who is very far away. If you are trying to talk to someone in trouble, or rather, to encourage them to talk to you, there is a useful kernel here which I hope might suggest ways in which you might approach them.

'A person is feeling suicidal. They cause an accident, deliberately. Why? I can't even begin. Another person dies. The charge is murder, not manslaughter. I decide I'm going to do the assessment with no doctors present.'

Without a great deal of experience, John's approach would be madness.

He continues, 'I sit them at a V-shape so eye contact is glancing. The nurse sits further away. Before we go in, I say to her, "I can't write anything but you're going to write, because the attention level that I need to give them is so huge it's almost painful." Imagine you are inaccessible to yourself. I've got to form a psychological bond to you. My concentration isn't going to waver for seventy-five minutes. I'm going to give you space to put yourself back together. You're going to be suicidal over what you've done, because it makes no more sense to you than it does to me. I *did* get an interview. It was the only time they spoke over the next few months. The pain . . .

'It's hugely tiring but I'm *slightly* intervening, offering you a little way back to the next stage of the story. I'm all invested in reaching you. There is no "me" left. Even though it's a nightmare for all concerned – they've got to go to jail, they have capacity – it's a good assessment.'

John's house is elegantly spare, lit by silvery winter sunlight pouring into the bare garden and through the large kitchen windows. He takes a book off the shelf – Cartier-Bresson's photographs. He shows me a famous image of the sculptor Alberto Giacometti, blurred, stepping between two of his sculptures, angular figures whose strides mirror Giacometti's own: or is it the other way around? We talk about the moment, the moment when self and other are in mirror exchange, when you could be the person in trouble or the person trying to help, and both of you are almost both at once. I ask John about helping people who may be longing not to exist, but who can be helped to avoid both death and detention. Again, we are talking about the more extreme situations, but there are echoes of these, and in John's approach, for anyone who has ever wished they could end it all. One in 5 people have suicidal thoughts, and 1 in 15 attempt it. All of us who know these thoughts are on a spectrum – it doesn't really matter where you cut it, we are suffering in the same deeply fundamental ways – and we can be helped by the same concepts, behaviours and strategies.

John says, 'I need *him* to help me not to detain him. Gradually he tells me things, things he's never told anyone. I have to be a guardian to these disclosures because in a way he's disclosing these things to himself. Do you know the Romanian philosopher Emil Cioran?

"Without the possibility of suicide I would have killed myself long ago." What this highlights is that the *idea* of suicide may be helping to keep the person alive by giving them a sense of control over the possibility of death.'

So if someone is chronically suicidal, this can be a strategy to cope with recurrent distress and the consequences of trauma. John knows it from both sides, having coped with it for a long time.

He cites psychologist and author Jesse Bering:

As for my own recurring compulsion to end my life, which flares up like a sore tooth at the whims of bad fortune, subsides for a while, yet always threatens to throb again, the types of problems that trigger these dangerous desires change over time [. . .] What made me suicidal as a teenager – the ever-looming prospect of being outed as gay in an intolerant small midwestern town – isn't what pushes those despairing buttons in me now [. . .] Other seemingly unsolvable problems seem to crop up as a matter of course.

John says, 'The thing about suicidality is people don't spot it. Indeed, it isn't easy to recognise if the person affected doesn't acknowledge it, which the pressures of everyday life often don't permit.'

Jesse Bering again:

What does a suicidal person look like? Me in that interview [. . .] I don't blame anyone for missing the signs.

What signs? Anyway, regrettably, I've done the same
[. . .] We're more intuitive than we give ourselves credit
for, but people aren't mind readers.

'You can't blame people for not spotting the signs,'
John says. 'What signs? A lot of this stuff doesn't come
with big placards. You want to be curious and inquisitive
about the people you love, but don't set the bar too high
and blame yourself for missing it. You wouldn't need as
many mental health professionals if people were listened to in the first place. You can't shake the person
until the truth falls out of them. It's a dialogue. So when
I am working with anyone who retains capacity and for
whom suicidality is a part of who they are, it is far better
not to try to forcibly take their "suicide card" away. You
focus on helping people get through today and tomorrow, rather than unrealistically, and at a bad time, demand
they give up on suicidality or be detained. All the more
so because, as psychiatrists such as Joel Paris have shown
us, we're unlikely to successfully "treat" chronic suicidality in hospital, and may actually make it worse. So you're
thinking, "Psychiatry is a risk for you. You've got to give
yourself the thirteenth, the fourteenth chance. Can you
make some sense of yourself without psychiatry?
Because if you can't, you're going to have to make sense
of psychiatry."'

What John is saying here is that the psychiatric system
as he knows it, both as a patient and a professional,
can do more harm than good. 'I'm not psychiatry's

handmaiden; I'm psychiatry's policeman,' he says. 'Often the shoulder I put my hand on is psychiatry's, to lead the psychiatrist gently away from the situation!

'Matt Simpson [an AMHP, like John] insisted on taking a highly distressed person whom he knew well out of seclusion. There were already two medical rec-ommendations for detention, but Matt used his previous knowledge of how to be with her to calm a situation which had been unwittingly exacerbated by unhelpful service responses. He phones the person's partner and takes her home, where the crisis team follow up. It looks crazy but it works – he *knows* this person. And he knows what he can do, so he knows what he *must* do. Matt's atti-tude is, "I'm not going to let them take you because I know that I can find an alternative to this well-intentioned overdose of psychiatry."

'Robert Lewis, author of national guidance about AMHP services, asked a service user what was the main thing he wanted from an AMHP. "The main thing I'm looking for is for you to give a shit!" That's an entirely reasonable benchmark, and needs to mean reaching the person in the way we assess. But sustained authenticity will have a psychological price that many professionals find too expensive, and you can't punish yourself by being totally present all the time. So your strategy of survival comes at a cost to those you see.'

This strikes me as particularly worth noting if you are looking out for someone, or looking after them. Fit your own oxygen mask first, as they say on aeroplanes. Attend to your own well-being as you attend to those around you. And remember, you are dealing with a patchwork system which does not work as well as it should, to put it mildly.

As John puts it, 'Mental health services are more disordered than the service user. You may get a high dose of professional anxiety when you hoped for reassurance – "We've got to make you fit what we think you're fit for!" You may have to fit the remit of existing services to get your needs met. And so you get chain referrals – people who don't fit are shunted from service to service because no one believes we can help you, but no one wants to say it. You are likely to be discharged from services, but if you are seen as "risky" and "disengaging", then detention may seem the only option.'

I am aware this is not a happy picture, but it seems useful to know that if you are experiencing this sort of treatment, you are not alone and it is not your fault.

Having been introduced to the background of how John and professionals like him think and work, we come to the crux: drawing on all of his experience, his insight and his knowledge, I want to know how John would advise the rest of us to help and talk to someone in distress.

John sits opposite me at his kitchen table, his face wrinkled with concentration. 'If someone's in trouble, and what you're doing or saying doesn't seem to be helping, you may think – is this about me? And too many of those self-doubting questions are *not* helpful. You've got to be as normal as possible.'

This seems so true and fundamental that it is worth noting this as a rule:

Rule 24: If someone close to you is in trouble you might think, is this about me? But the question is not helpful; you've got to be as normal as possible.

'You can have an encounter where there are two conversations going on,' John says. 'One spoken, one unspoken. Through what we say we can show something *beyond* what we're saying. We show our understanding. If I went for the jugular of the problem you'd find it incredibly difficult. So we have to gently find a space. In the beginning was the deed, as Goethe said. There's stuff that has to come before – to find the words that matter, you have to create the space and the meaning. For example, one of my colleagues on an outreach team was asked how he could achieve such trust. It was because he played pool with the person! It created a rhythm for the conversation.

'I worked with someone who had psychotic depression. He had killed his wife and tried to kill himself. I saw him many, many times in the next year. We went walking in the country when he was on leave from the ward. I feel the pace that he's walking and I walk at exactly that pace. I ask a question with a few words. It's not silence between us because we keep on walking. The rhythm of our steps holds things together until he is ready to speak. So it can be about actually doing something together, not having a chat, because there will be *words*, and they're not necessarily the right words. Or the words may be few but the manner of your presence speaks deeply to the person.

'How does love show itself most effectively? Find something that shows that. Somewhere you've walked, somewhere you drive to. A song. A rhythm of you being together, however slow or however inconspicuous. It's about finding the place, in so many ways.'

As he speaks, I begin to understand that John teaches a kind of gentle obliqueness – a coming in from the side, emotionally, physically, mentally.

'Suppose you ask me, "Why are you doing such and such a thing?" To reply to that I've got to say, "I feel shit," or, "I've got no energy." So instead you look for something, however tiny, with a positive in it. You don't demand, confront – instead, you just turn up. You say, "Let's go for a walk." It's about unthreatening directness. You're offering to share something. Not caring is, "I don't do that, but *you* should go off and do it."

'Say alcohol is not very good for you, and you're drinking too much, but my having a drink with you might not be the worst thing – for a friend, not as an AMHP! You're looking for the knowledge of what is the best of them, and you've got to find that in an unthreatening way. A modicum of self-disclosure in a personal relationship is extremely powerful. These are the times when skilled friends and family say, "Well, yes, me and your dad were going to split up but . . ."

'So to a seventeen-year-old you're *listening*. You're sharing a conversation – not piling on loads of self-disclosure, but information in conversation. If I don't give you anything, then I'm not trying hard enough.'

Like a rapidly growing number of professionals, John believes that the network approach taken by Open Dialogue is key.

As he puts it, 'Knowing *who* is close. You can do something helpful by getting someone in touch with the right person to unburden themselves to, even if you're not that person.'

It strikes me that this all makes great sense – but supposing you love that person, supposing you are desperate to help them, supposing that desperation is infusing the way you approach them and your time together. How do you make this work with someone you love, when your love is expressing itself as anxiety, frustration, gnawing worry?

'The thing to think is, "I can't promise not to be judgemental because I care about you, but I'm going to keep my judgemental nature in check because you have options." The war won't be won today. It's all about maximising the chances – not of sorting everything out in this conversation, but that there *will be* conversations two, three, four and five. An overdose of truth isn't going to be the most helpful thing. Find the right dose of truth. For a harsh dose of truth, you may only need 2mg of that! Show what it means to be honest. Have humility. How are you going to get yourself to their level? Because you can't be up *there* [he holds his hand above his head], can you, while they're down here?'

John uses variations of the same approach – one you might take with someone who is anxious, worried, depressed or self-doubting – with people who are breaking down, subject to delusions, paranoia or flights of ideas.

'Well, what are they saying? It's all in the emotions and the tone in which they're telling the story. Their emotion is somewhere else – with spies or aliens – but you've shown you've heard it. Sometimes you *so* don't have the answers, and you're *so* bewildered by them not being themselves, that all you can be is with them.

'A friend of mine who is expert in Ancient Greek was caring for a retired professor of classics who had developed dementia. The professor's grandchild had brought him a toy windmill and put it on his window sill. The professor was disturbed by it, and fearful – what is that? And my friend said, "Don't worry, Professor, it's just a *techne*," – in Greek, a machine that does a job of work, hoping to convey by that single Greek word that, whatever it was, it was a thing made with art, craft, skill. And that was it – it was fine, a tailored gesture of reassurance. So what you're looking for is the language of their soul. It's not as hard as it sounds – it's the rhythm of their own self-soothing.

'So if you are with someone with anxiety, don't keep feeding that message, that they're anxious and you're anxious. Ease off. Feel how close you can get without provoking it. One sentence, one acknowledgement can be key. And a sense of humour! There's a Penelope Fitzgerald character who drives a hundred miles expressly to say nothing to his dearest friend. But he turns up.* The outcomes are always best when there's a sense of humour.'

> **Rule 25: To help someone in trouble, keep turning up, keep listening, and know that the most important thing is the relationship between you, and your ongoing conversation. Go easy on yourself, and them.**

John says, 'Suppose you've got a nineteen-year-old university student and something has gone wrong. Suppose Mum turns up on the doorstep. She doesn't have to say much. That she turns up means she *recognises* something's wrong.'

Later, as John drives me back to the station, he talks about his life. He studied philosophy at Swansea, and later social work at Exeter. He has been detained a number of times. During his thirties he had a period of homelessness.

'I became a tramp, wandering from place to place,' he

---

* In Penelope Fitzgerald's novel *The Bookshop*: 'Even Lord Gosfield was touched, though he had said nothing all evening, and had in fact driven the hundred-odd miles expressly to say nothing in the company of his old friend Bruno.'

says. For a lot of his life he has felt himself 'half in love with death'.

He has learned to cope with suicidality and anxiety.

'Sometimes I've found myself nearly vomiting with fear at the start of every working day – but I know I can cope with that. And if you've felt that, you can help people,' he says, with a look of great gentleness, 'provided that you listen. In helping lies the possibility of your own recovery. You have to be open about these things, and honest. And keep moving along in a positive direction!'

We talk about the necessity of being comfortable with uncertainty – the key to so much of the journey, to recovery, to healing; the key to all journeys, perhaps, and especially to the British transport system. As usual, the trains have been all over the place all day: ice, strikes, signal failure.

At the station there is a very friendly woman at the barrier. Should I go early to Crewe and find my way home the long way around? 'Yes,' she says, 'I would, the way things have been going.' Does it matter about my pre-booked ticket for a later train? 'No!' she smiles. 'Today we have cross-acceptance.'

The lady at the barrier seemed, most miraculously, to sum up so much of what John says. Cross-acceptance. Accept where they are, and who they are, at the moment, and know that underneath the moment, and stretching out ahead, are many more, which can be very different and much better.

To help someone, do not come in head-on. Remember the oblique angle – just being with them can be as powerful as anything. Be as normal as possible. Do not let words get in the way. Do not let time get in the way. Precipitate speech can obscure what needs to be shared: this might be a peaceful exchange in near silence, until they are ready to talk. Find ways to be together in a happy place. Accept that this is a process, never a final battle. Give unlimited chances. Be tolerant of situations which seem to be going nowhere; you are together, you are in exchange, the person is frightened of their situation, not you. It can come out, given time, especially if your anxiety about them isn't catching. When appropriate, give all your attention. When appropriate, share your uncertainty.

Remember John's tools: a modicum of self-disclosure can be very powerful; listening is all; being able to share the space with someone, and hold the hope in it, is to give a huge gift.

'How does love show itself most effectively?' John asked. And he answered it: 'You're looking for the knowledge of what is the best of them.' If you can listen to, speak with and be alongside that best of them, you are doing something wonderful.

19. Worlds of hope

In order to bring about the world we want to live in, the world we want our children and grandchildren to live in, we have first to imagine it, and then to work backwards, step by step, day by day, to the present. This will give us a map to follow, a real traveller's guide, for all of us who travel through the vicissitudes of the strange and difficult and miraculous country that is life in the world.

The truth is that despite decades of little progress in terms of new medications, and the protracted under-funding of services, resulting in chronic waiting times and abominable shortages of nursing staff, beds, therapists, psychiatrists and modern hospitals, we *are* on our way towards better understanding and better treating mental health.

Remember the *Diagnostic and Statistical Manual of Mental Disorders* from Chapter 2 ('Who owns the words?'). The *DSM*-influenced practice of diagnosing sufferers according to checklists and assigning us conditions, as if putting us into boxes, is being questioned, and it is waning. For decades, we suffered as individuals but we were treated as categories: there is a wide and spreading acknowledgement that no one's condition is quite the same as anyone else's. There is a broadening comprehension, among clinicians and sufferers, that while diagnosis can bring life-changing benefits, the language of categorisation may not be useful or helpful to an individual.

As the demand for therapy grows, more and more people are choosing to train or retrain as therapists. Even if we cannot afford or easily access therapy, therapy's lessons are being absorbed across society: we know that exercise, meaningful activity, sleep, self-care, nutrition, being open about our feelings and asking for help – whether we ask it of our employers, our institutions, our families, our friends or our networks – can make huge differences.

As the CHIME framework becomes more widely known we will better understand that connection, hope, identity, meaning and empowerment offer us paths to recovery. One of the consequences of the Covid pandemic is a resounding assault on stigma: lockdowns taught us that mental health is part of all human lives, and showed us how we can maintain and support it. The young are less likely to feel trapped and silenced by fear of stigma than their parents were. There is more information available, and more ways to connect with fellow sufferers, than ever before. We now know that we need each other, we need activity, we need the outdoors, we need to feel heard and seen, and we need to feel that we can make a contribution.

One of the most exciting and illuminating experiences for me in researching and writing this book has been the discovery, introduced to me by Professor Mike Slade, of post-traumatic growth. Like most people, I had never heard of it; and knowing about it is the first stage of experiencing it. Imagine going to your GP, suffering from anxiety or depression. Your GP talks you through options for treatment and coping strategies. And then they say, 'Are you ready for some really good news?'

You surely are.

'Right, you have been going through and coping with a horribly hard time for very good reasons – the situation you find yourself in would produce anxiety and depression in pretty well anyone. You are normal, and your responses, your feelings, may feel like hell but they are normal and healthy. And now the really good news. You are about to experience post-traumatic growth. Researchers in America who identified this phenomenon found that 89 per cent of people who experienced significant trauma, including illness, bereavement and shattering life events like relationship breakdown, accidents and the terrible hardships caused by war or displacement, experience post-traumatic growth.

'You are likely to find that you experience greater appreciation for life and a strengthening of close relationships. You are likely to become more compassionate, more altruistic and more resilient. You may find that you see more possibilities and purpose in your life. You are likely to gain a greater appreciation of your personal strengths, along with a greater sense of how to use them. Do not be surprised if you develop a stronger spiritual sense of your place and purpose in the world, and grow creatively. How do you feel now?'

Had my GP or psychiatrist said this to me, I would have left the appointment filled with a delighted sense of hope and purpose. And thanks to the expectancy effect, shown in countless placebo trials, whereby people who believe they are going to receive a benefit do indeed experience that benefit, I would be tremendously more likely to be stepping out into a life of post-traumatic growth. If an authoritative source like a doctor or psychiatrist – or, more commonly, one of the mental health websites that comes up first on Google – tells you that you can expect a life of suffering, your morale, your motivation to make changes and your sense of agency all take a plunge. The opposite is also true. *Everyone* who suffers needs to know about post-traumatic growth; every doctor and psychiatrist could – and, we can only hope, will – become familiar with it in the years to come.

Another reason for hope is that many of us with lived experience of mental health crises are now putting our experiences to work for others and ourselves, in defiance of stigma. I interviewed Jonny Ward, a psychotherapist, mental health trainer and watch manager at one of the busier fire services in the country. Jonny was fighting fires and rescuing people while suffering and hiding attacks of acute anxiety. The single biggest change in his mental health, he told me, was the day he went into work and told his colleagues, including the team he was tasked to lead into mortal danger, that he suffered from anxiety.

'How was that?' I asked.

'The most liberating experience I've ever had in my life,' Jonny replied. 'And I'm so grateful.'

His managers, his colleagues and his team all accepted what he told them and were untroubled by it. They respected him for telling them about his condition, and his firefighters followed him into battle with the fires with even more confidence. The day he told them about his struggles with anxiety, deliberately confronting and realising what had become a crippling fear of being found out, felt, he said, 'Like I took a rucksack off.' He describes the consequence of admitting, confronting and sharing his feelings as, 'Owning my world.'

Jonny's story is an inspiring example of post-traumatic growth: from being a man with a terrible secret and a crippling condition, he now trains teams and individuals in ways of coping with anxiety, and ways of growing through it. The more readily we are able to be frank and open with ourselves and others about the experience of carrying our own rucksacks, the easier and the sooner we will be able to shed them, and the closer we will come to owning our own worlds.

I hope this book has helped you to identify helpful ways of thinking about and addressing your mental health, or that of someone you are worried about. And I hope, pray and expect that in the coming years and decades the ways in which we understand and treat mental health will be utterly and comprehensively different from how our systems work now.

To bring about a better world, we must be able to imagine and see it.

Imagine no stigma attaches to anyone with anxiety or depression or psychosis, because these come to be seen (as they already are by the most progressive clinicians and therapists) as explicable and reasonable responses to an individual's experiences, situation and circumstances.

Imagine our children are taught from an early age how to recognise the signs of mental distress, and to understand them as normal parts of life, which do not mark you out in any way – these are the logical and sensitive reactions of a sensitive, thoughtful, feeling person.

Imagine our children live in areas where they have instant access to a range of therapies – from talking, to walking, to art. Imagine their towns and cities, their offices and institutions are constructed and run with the well-being of the inhabitants and occupants first, and the profits of corporations second.

Imagine a system in which everyone has on-demand access to trauma therapy, EMDR and Open Dialogue. Imagine these are the first, the front-line treatments, and medication the second, or final: the fallback.

Imagine better drugs, with fewer side effects, prescribed by clinicians who understand them, and who can explain what they do and do not know about them, and how their benefits are best realised; they give you a solid place to stand, a place in which you can make changes.

Imagine more psychiatrists with a greater range of tools at their disposal – from access to therapists, to social prescribing. Psychiatrists who can give the care which so many long to give: offering regular appointments to the same patients. Psychiatrists whose wisdom, humility and willingness to admit uncertainty make them partners in their patients' treatments, rather than random and hurried interveners.

Imagine an entire system based on an empowering recovery model, in which signs of difficulty are taken as a trigger for helpful and healing interventions, rather than the current model, in which, too often, difficulty and distress lead to stigmatising categorisation, and (many) diagnoses lead to despair.

Imagine a world where no one is ever again given a ghettoising, cruel label; where phrases like 'personality disorder' are never heard again in a punitive or denigrating context, and only used, of themselves, by those who might find them useful and empowering. Imagine all the harm that clumsy diagnostic categories have done being apologised for, and corrected.

Imagine mental hospitals and psychiatric wards where you would be glad to spend time yourself, if you needed a break; wards where well-paid, well-trained, well-led, well-motivated staff create a compassionate therapeutic environment; places where you can have as much therapy of the kind that most helps you as you require; places where gardening, art, horticulture, hydrotherapy and music therapy are available daily.

Most fundamentally of all, imagine that your first contact with a GP or specialist did not lead to you being categorised as someone with some mysterious fault or 'chemical imbalance' who is now doomed to a life of managing a stigmatising 'condition', with only little help, less understanding and sporadic, if any, support. Imagine leaving that first appointment with a new perspective: there is nothing fundamentally 'wrong' with you. You are a sensitive human being who is reacting to your story and your circumstances as sensitive people do. No one else has what you have, but millions have something like it. You are not going to spend the rest of your life plagued by mental illness, for 'diseases' of the mind are not diseases at all, merely concepts. You are on a journey of recovery and post-traumatic growth which has started today. You can and should come out of this a wiser, better, even stronger person, with even more to give.

All this is possible, because all of it is happening somewhere, right now. There is a better world around us and ahead of us. We can and we must fight to bring it about.

We can demand that NHS trusts in our area invest in treatments which have been unequivocally shown to work, like Open Dialogue and EMDR.

We can write to our MPs and local government chief executives asking for more art therapists, for more NHS clinical psychologists, for more psychiatrists, for shorter waiting lists and more appointments.

We could make a point of voting for politicians who are committed to defending and increasing NHS spending on mental health.

We can alert the press and the public whenever we find anything in the system which is unhelpful, obstructive or harmful.

We can campaign against stigma by educating the young: we could teach them that mental health and well-being are natural parts of this life, and not to be unduly feared, and not to be looked down upon, or hidden, or fled from.

We could help them further by teaching them simple well-being techniques, mentally healthy behaviours and activities, and by giving young people an unthreatening vocabulary with which to understand and identify mental health problems. (Imagine the difference it would make if every fifteen-year-old had a clear understanding of post-traumatic growth, for example, and if every eighteen-year-old could explain what the CHIME framework is, and how it has been shown to work.)

We can support people like Mike Slade in their efforts to swing our outdated and creaking system towards a progressive and healing recovery model.

We can keep talking, posting, sharing and supporting one another, in the determined knowledge that we have made great progress in mental health, and that we will, as sure as humans were born to make things, make a great deal more.

We can never give up.

Afterword

And there is just one more thing I would say to anyone I loved who was in trouble, and which I would like to say to you, or to the person you are worried about.

We know it can be a miserable hell, to feel trapped in your mind and body by feelings and fears and guilts and nightmares and miserable reactions, and that grey dragging hopelessness you feel you cannot control.

When it happens to me I try to ask myself: When was the last time I laughed – really, roaringly laughed? When did I last hug someone and tell them I loved them? And when did someone last hug me, and say that to me? When was the last time I kissed someone I love? When was the last time I walked in a beautiful place? When was the last time I was not thinking about anything except where I was, and about the moments of the world around me? When was the last time my whole soul seemed to sing with joy at the beauty of the world, and the infinite goodness in it? When was the last time I did someone a kindness? When did I last do a good piece of work? When did I last see great art, hear great music, watch great theatre or film? When was the last time a book took me far away? When was the last time I was able to forget myself, because I was concentrating completely on helping someone else? When was the last time I swam in the sea, or danced, or sang, or cooked something delicious, or used my hands for a job of good work, or treated someone, or really looked after someone, or tried something new, or saw a new horizon, or walked in an entirely new place?

When did I last feel that I was standing in a world and a life which have been given to me, as I have been given to them?

The answer, in my darkest periods, is often: *Ages*, or, *So long ago I can't remember.*

And the conclusions I draw from this are:

a. I need to do some or all of these things again, as soon as I can.
b. Anyone would feel worse for the lack of them, and anyone will feel better for them, and when they come they will be a signal I am healing, and part of my healing.
c. Most importantly – they will come again, and I will hold on until they do because they WILL come again. They will. They will. *They will.*

20. The rules

Rule 1: No one else has what I have.

Rule 2: I call it whatever is most helpful to me.

Rule 3: I am not my suffering; I am not my symptoms.

Rule 4: No website can know me better than I can know myself.

Rule 5: Madness is in all of us, and the world is surely mad.

Rule 6: You are normal, and likely not especially different to anyone else. You feel different because pressure, trauma, unhappiness, or something in your life or history, is making you feel and act in certain ways. Anyone in your position would feel and act the same way.

Rule 7: Medication can be a lifesaver, but most psychiatric medication can only treat symptoms, not causes.

Rule 8: We suffer as individuals, but we are treated as categories. You are dealing with an overloaded, underfunded and creaky system. Insist on your treatment being as individual as possible.

Rule 9: Accessing what you need when you need it will be work, perhaps hard and frustrating work. But know the help is out there.

Rule 10: The Addiction Monster, as some therapists call it, is infinitely beatable. It feeds on silence and shame – so speak out. It feeds on solitude – so find a peer supporter. It feeds on inertia – so act.

Rule 11: A breakdown is saying, you cannot do this any more; you need to stop and you need to reset. As such, a breakdown is the first step on a journey of healing and recovery. It is *not* a sign that there is anything fundamentally wrong with you.

Rule 12: If you are certain that someone you care about needs help, and you find yourself fighting to get it for them, use the most forceful and unambiguous language: fight in the terms the system understands.

Rule 13: The idea that 'they', the 'normal', are over there, in their great successful majority, and that 'we', the sufferers, are over here, in our particular personal torment, is an illusion.

Rule 14: If nothing else works, if you really have tried everything else, if you are in need of a last resort, then that is what medication is there for.

Rule 15: If you are offered a medication, always ask why you are being offered it. Ask what else you could take instead of this, i.e. why this one, why now?

Rule 16: Never be embarrassed to be full and frank about the details and dimensions of your symptoms, physical and mental. Do not be 'British' about suffering. Do not try to 'Grin and Bear It'. Do not try to 'Keep Calm and Carry On'.

Rule 17: Medication can give you a place to stand: solid mental ground and stabilised emotions. Use that solid ground to make the changes that will make a long-term difference.

Rule 18: We all carry our child selves inside us. Shutting down that child's pain, or blocking it out, or blaming yourself for the feelings it produces, are not the right responses. That child needs love, help, hearing and care. That child needs therapy.

Rule 19: You are going to do most of your own healing, and for that you need a strong sense of self. There are ways of building up that sense (this book is full of them). Get to it.

Rule 20: What happens to you is not about anyone else's narrative. It's about yours. Do not tell yourself a story which dooms you to suffering. Do the work you need to live and tell a story of recovery.

Rule 21: To help yourself, help others.

Rule 22: To help someone who is in trouble, 'I believe you will find your way through this and I am here to help you find it,' is more effective than, 'This is the way to get better.'

Rule 23: There *is* an established and proven route to recovery – it is called the CHIME framework. If you follow it, you will maximise your chances of recovery. If you are helping someone, remember it is not your job to fix them; your job is to support and believe in their power to help themselves.

Rule 24: If someone close to you is in trouble you might think, is this about me? But the question is not helpful; you've got to be as normal as possible.

Rule 25: To help someone in trouble, keep turning up, keep listening, and know that the most important thing is the relationship between you, and your ongoing conversation. Go easy on yourself, and them.

Acknowledgements

This book is written in tribute and in gratitude to all those working for a radically happier and more effectively caring world, and in particular admiration for the remarkable people whose advice, ideas and passionate professionalism I have aimed to describe here. Any error or infelicity is mine alone. Great thanks to Yasmin Ishaq, John Mitchell, Professor Mike Slade, Juliet Shepherd, Sue Holmes, Moyra Bentley, Dr Kate Kerr, Ellen Sieg, Tamara Moon, Dr Swapnil Gupta and Professor Femi Oyebode.

The writing ran alongside the making of the first series of *Is Psychiatry Working?*, commissioned and kindly guided for BBC Radio 4 by Mohit Bakaya and Dan Clarke, expertly edited by Clare Fordham, brilliantly and tirelessly produced by Emma Close, co-hosted (and magnificently elevated!) by Professor Femi Oyebode. My huge thanks to you all. It is a complete pleasure and an education to work with you, dear Emma and dear Femi: you make finding our ways through the labyrinths of the brain, the BBC and the mental health system a true joy. Thank you.

Thank you to Sarah Hamilton, Clare-Marie Heaney and Ewan Hilton at Platfform, Brigid Bowen and Benna Waites at Compassionate Mental Health, Professor

Felice Jacka at the Food & Mood Centre, Professor Catherine Harmer at the Psychopharmacology and Emotional Research Lab, Robert Whitaker at Mad in America, Jonny Ward at The Anxious Firefighter, Leah Charles-King, António Ferreira at Hear Me Speak, Dr Chloe Beale and Clare Shaw. I am deeply grateful for your time, trouble and frankness.

Huge thanks to Olivia Kumar and to Zoë Waldie, my most wonderful and perspicacious agent, at Rogers, Coleridge and White. You two are just *the* most kind, patient, warm and brilliant team: I am ever and delightedly in your debt.

Thank you, especially, to Connor Brown at Viking, for seeing this book so clearly, believing in it so brightly and editing it so skilfully and patiently. Great thanks to Shân Morley Jones for your model copy edit and wonderful encouragement.

My own journey owes everything to the love, support and beautiful friendship of Merlin and Anna Rose Hughes, Roger Couhig, Chris Kenyon, Robin Jenkins, Graham Da Gama Howells, Kevin Bohnert, Niall Griffiths, Debs Jones, Natalie Haynes, Robert Macfarlane, Dan Richards, Gareth Gavin, Kaye Mitchell, Jeremy Grange, Carole Green, Andy Fell, Jodie Bond, Mo Bakaya, Rob Ketteridge, Lawrence Pollard, Allegra McIlroy, Alison Finch, Richard Coles, Peter Florence, Becky Shaw, Gracie and Adrian Cooper, Ben Myers, Rozie Kelly and Zaffar Kunial. Thank you, you great lights.

ACKNOWLEDGEMENTS

To my family and patchwork family – Rebecca, Jenny, Emma and Chris Shooter, Robin Tetlow-Shooter, Doug and Ellie Field, Jeff Young, Scott and Gail Tetlow, Anthea Robinson, Roy, Sarah and Cindy Clare, Esther Maylor, Aubrey Shooter Clare (darling Bug!), Alexander and Sally Clare – my love and thanks forever.

Notes

2. *Who owns the words? (And why they matter)*

p. 13 **He cites a 2007 study . . . which concludes**: Huxley,
N. & Baldessarini, R. J. 2007. 'Disability and its treatment in
bipolar disorder patients'. *Bipolar Disorders*, 9 (1-2), 183–96.

3. *What I've got: Diagnosis (just for you)*

p. 24 **Data emerging from both academic centers and
from public and private outpatient facilities indicate**: Perugi, G. et al. 2015. 'Cyclothymia reloaded: A
reappraisal of the most misconceived affective disorder'.
Journal of Affective Disorders, 183, 119–33.

9. *Common maladies: Dope and hope*

p. 98 **A landmark study funded by the Economic and
Social Research Council**: The COVID Social Mobility
& Opportunities Study (COSMO), published in Novem-
ber 2022.

p. 110 **The brain continues to develop through childhood and adolescence**: Kate Kellaway, 'Sarah-Jayne Blakemore: "It is, strangely, acceptable to mock and demonise teenagers"'. *Observer*, 25 March 2018.

p. 113 **The Canigma website offers this excellent list of recommendations**: Lassalle's piece about side effects, which every dope smoker should read, is here: https://cannigma.com/treatment/how-to-mitigate-the-side-effects-of-cannabis/.

10. Crisis

p. 136 **Physical symptoms may include**: https://www.nhsinform.scot/illnesses-and-conditions/mental-health/anxiety/.

p. 139 **In 2019, I interviewed a former patient at the Broadoak Unit**: Public findings concerning the unit include https://www.jacksonlees.co.uk/broudiejackson-canter/jury-finds-failings-care-broadoak-unit; and also https://www.bbc.co.uk/news/uk-england-merseyside-36709125.

p. 141 **At the time of writing people can be detained for**: Mental Health Act 1983. See https://www.legislation.gov.uk/ukpga/1983/20/part/II/crossheading/procedure-for-hospital-admission?view=plain.

p. 141 **But researchers, NHS directors and policymakers are proposing**: UK Government: Reforming the Mental Health Act white paper, August 2021.

11. Medication: Background and basics

p. 156 **A review by researchers at University College London**: Moncrieff, J. et al. 2023. 'The serotonin theory of depression: a systematic umbrella review of the evidence'. *Molecular Psychiatry*, 28, 3243–56.

p. 157 **'Our view is that patients should not be told'**: Julia Robinson, 'The serotonin theory of depression: how the media got it all wrong'. *Pharmaceutical Journal*, 31 August 2022.

p. 167 **They concluded that this popular drug was**: Barbui, C., Furukawa, T. A. & Cipriani, A. 2008. 'Effectiveness of paroxetine in the treatment of acute major depression in adults: a systematic re-examination of published and unpublished data from randomized trials'. *Canadian Medical Association Journal*, 178 (3), 296–305.

p. 169 **Overall, a balanced appraisal of the effectiveness of medication**: Mike Slade. 2009. *Personal Recovery and Mental Illness: A Guide for Mental Health Professionals*. New York, NY: Cambridge University Press, pp. 66–7.

p. 170 **Some patients will take medication as suggested by the prescriber**: ibid., p. 68.

14. The self-work of recovery

p. 221 **This story was published . . . and picked up by a newspaper**: See Rhys Blakely, 'Acts of kindness "can be better than therapy" for depression and anxiety'. *The Times*, 11 January 2023.

p. 222 **Researchers looked at people who helped others during the Hurricane Sandy disaster in the US**: Hu, T. Y. et al. 2016. 'Helping others, warming yourself: Altruistic behaviors increase warmth feelings of the ambient environment'. *Frontiers in Psychology*, 7, article 1349.

p. 222 **A second study confirmed the first**: Feng, L. & Guo, Q. 2016. 'Beneficial effect of altruism on well-being among Chinese college students: The role of self-esteem and family socioeconomic status'. *Journal of Social Service Research*, November, 1–16.

p. 228 **So no, there isn't that kind of evidence**: Verghese, A. 2008. 'Spirituality and Mental Health'. *Indian Journal of Psychiatry*, 50 (4), 233–7; Goncalves, J. P. B. et al. 2015. 'Religious and spiritual interventions in mental health care: a systematic review and meta-analysis of randomized controlled clinical trials'. *Psychological Medicine*, 45 (14), 2937–49.

15. Bouncing back better: Post-traumatic growth

p. 238 **It just creates a social milieu that leads to wholly different trajectories**: A comprehensive 2014 report into peer supporter-run services by the Kites Trust in New Zealand found that people treated in Key We Way had the highest regard for the institution, praising every aspect of the care they received. They had two suggestions for improvement: 1) Popularity of the service meant they could not stay as long as they would have liked; 2) They felt the staff, the peer support workers, should be paid more.

16. On the ward

p. 250 **In February 2023 the *Nursing Times* reported**: Megan Ford, 'Staffing "significant barrier" to improving mental health services'. *Nursing Times*, 9 February 2023.

p. 251 **In July 2023 the Public Accounts Committee published a report**: UK Parliament Committees. 'Concerning pressures on NHS mental health staff causing vicious cycle of staff shortages'. 21 July 2023.

p. 251 **Research by the British Medical Association**: See https://www.bma.org.uk/news-and-opinion/further-than-ever.

p. 252 **In 2023, the mental health charity Mind listed recent scandals**: News and campaigns. 'More than a third of adults lack confidence in mental health hospitals after string of scandals'. 20 June 2023.

p. 253 **a report by NHS Providers, which represents NHS trusts**:https://nhsproviders.org/news-blogs/news/patient-safety-standards-at-risk-while-majority-of-mental-health-trusts-do-not-have-access-to-the-funding-they-need-to-address-urgent-repairs-and-upgrade-services.

p. 253 **Writing to Members of Parliament in 2022 . . . Dr Adrian James, said**: Andrew Gregory, 'Call for six new mental health hospitals in England as buildings "crumble away"'. *Guardian*, 8 February 2022.

p. 256 **One obvious reason that 1.5 million people are on NHS waiting lists**: Shaun Lintern. 'More than one million waiting for mental health treatment with one in 10 doctor posts empty'. *Independent*, 7 October 2021.

p. 277 **In 2023, West Lane Hospital in Middlesbrough was found to be**: Poppy Kennedy, 'Inside "chaotic and unsafe" West Lane Hospital where teens took own lives as health chiefs missed "red flags"'. *Teesside News*, 21 March 2023.

17. Healing in action: Art therapy

p. 283 **National Alliance on Mental Illness in the US puts partial or full recovery from serious mental illness at 65 per cent**: Larry Davidson and Katherine Ponte. 'Serious mental illness recovery: The basics'. NAMI, 11 August 2021.

p. 283 **The NHS calculates that 49.3 per cent of people suffering from anxiety or depression**: https://www.england.nhs.uk/2018/02/mental-illness-recovery/.

p. 300 **studies in the US found that art therapy improved symptoms**: Emblad, S. Y. M. & Mukaetova-Ladinska, E. B. 2021. 'Creative art therapy as a non-pharmacological intervention for dementia: A systematic review'. *Journal of Alzheimer's Disease Reports*, 5 (1), 353–64.

p. 300 **in healthy volunteers whose stress levels were measured by cortisol levels**: Kaimal, G., Ray, K. &

Muniz, J. 2016. 'Reduction of cortisol levels and partici-pants' responses following art making'. *Art Therapy*, 33 (2), 74–80.

p. 300 **At Drexel University in the US, researchers found**: https://drexel.edu/news/archive/2017/june/making-art-activates-brains-reward-pathways.

18. How to talk to someone in trouble

p. 314 **As for my own recurring compulsion to end my life**: Jesse Bering. 2018. *A Very Human Ending: How Suicide Haunts Our Species*. London: Penguin, pp. 3–4.

p. 314 **What does a suicidal person look like?**: ibid., pp. 11–13.

p. 315 **All the more so because, as psychiatrists such as Joel Paris have shown us**: Joel Paris. 2023. *Half in Love with Death: Managing the Chronically Suicidal Patient*. 2nd Edition. London: Routledge.

p. 316 **Robert Lewis, author of national guidance about AMHP services**: Lewis, R., Linde, K. & Trewin, M. 2020. *Approved Mental Health Professional (AMHP) National Service Standards*. DHSC. Available at: https://www.hee.nhs.uk/sites/default/files/documents/National%20AMHP%20Service%20Standards.pdf.

p. 322 **There's a Penelope Fitzgerald character who drives a hundred miles**: Penelope Fitzgerald. 1978. *The Bookshop*. London: Gerald Duckworth & Co, p. 28.

19. Worlds of hope

p. 327 **Researchers in America who identified this phe-nomenon:** Tedeschi, R. G. & Calhoun, L. G. 2004. Target Article: 'Posttraumatic growth: Conceptual foundations and empirical evidence'. *Psychological Inquiry* 15 (1), 1–18.

Index

Moon, Tamara 143, 144,
    148–50, 269
Morgan-Grenville, Gerard 206
MRI studies 10, 11, 11*n*,
    119
Murray, Sir Robin 107

NA (Narcotics Anonymous)
    115–25
National Alliance on Mental
    Illness 283
network approach 320
Newson, Dr Louise 95
National Health Service
    (NHS) xiii, 10, 18, 19, 29,
    55, 57, 75, 76, 85, 91–2,
    100, 127, 133–48, 175,
    192, 193, 194, 250–51,
    253, 256, 333
    GPs *see* GP
    Improving Access to
        Psychological Therapies
        (IAPT) *see* Improving
        Access to Psychological
        Therapies (IAPT), NHS
    NHS Talking Therapies *see*
        NHS Talking Therapies
    Trusts *see individual trust name*
NHS Talking Therapies
    88–91, 92–3, 152. *See also*
    Improving Access to
    Psychological Therapies
    (IAPT), NHS

NICE guidelines 184
Niche Health 278
No More Panic 90
Nursing Times 250
Nurturers 205

Oakley, Mark 100
obliqueness, gentle 319, 324
obsessive-compulsive disorder
    (OCD) 135, 215
OCD Action 90
Open Dialogue xx, 50–84,
    124, 320, 322,
    330, 332
Oyebode, Femi xix, 10
over-resilience 128

panic disorder 135
Panorama (television
    programme) 139, 253,
    277, 278
Paris, Joel 315
Parliamentary and Health
    Service Ombudsman
    274, 275, 276, 279, 281
paroxetine 167
Peacock, Angie 163
peer support 59–60, 62,
    63, 64, 65, 66, 67, 79, 80,
    123–4, 223, 235, 238
personalised approach/
    treatment xiv, xviii, 3, 4,
    8, 15–16, 171

Vita Health Group 89
voices, hearing 35, 36, 38, 76

waiting times 91–2, 325
ward, psychiatric 50, 65, 68, 77,
    142, 151, 235, 238,
    246–81, 292, 304, 305,
    318, 331
Ward, Jonny 328–9
West Lane Hospital,
    Middlesbrough 277–8
Western medicine 128
What Really Matters 100
Whitaker, Robert 12–13
Whitwell, David 169
Wilmington Healthcare 76

winter blues xx, 2, 5–6, 15, 16,
    23, 25, 33, 36, 55, 82,
    212–13. *See also* Seasonal
    Affective Disorder (SAD)
Wise Figures and Protectors
    205–6
women 77, 93, 95, 196, 205
work, return to 13, 51, 76, 161,
    235–6
World Health Organisation
    167

young people 29–31, 90,
    97–114, 159, 161–2, 164,
    172–3, 247–8, 272–3, 326,
    333